Hospital Infection Control for Nurses

Peter Meers

Formerly Associate Professor
Microbiology Department
National University of Singapore and
One time Director
Division of Hospital Infection
Central Public Health Laboratory
Colindale, London, UK

Wendy Jacobsen

Infection Control Nurse
National University Hospital
Singapore

and

Madeleine McPherson

Infection Control Nurse
Fremantle Hospital
Western Australia

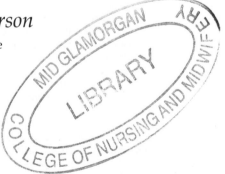

CHAPMAN & HALL

London · Glasgow · New York · Tokyo · Melbourne · Madras

Published by Chapman & Hall, 2-6 Boundary Row,
London SE1 8HN, UK

Chapman & Hall, 2-6 Boundary Row, London SE1 8HN, UK

Blackie Academic & Professional, Wester Cleddens Road,
Bishopbriggs, Glasgow G64 2NZ, UK

Chapman & Hall Inc., One Penn Plaza, 41st Floor, New York
NY 10119, USA

Chapman & Hall Japan, Thomson Publishing Japan, Hirakawacho
Nemoto Building, 6F, 1-7-11 Hirakawa-cho, Chiyoda-ku, Tokyo 102,
Japan

Chapman & Hall Australia, Thomas Nelson Australia, 102 Dodds
Street, South Melbourne, Victoria 3205, Australia

Chapman & Hall India, R. Seshadri, 32 Second Main Road, CIT East,
Madras 600 035, India

First edition 1992
Reprinted 1994

© 1992 Chapman & Hall

Typeset in 10/12pt Palatino by Excel Typesetters Company,
Hong Kong
Printed in Great Britain by Page Bros, Norwich

ISBN 0 412 47820 6   1 56593 060 6 (USA)

A catalogue record for this book is available from the British Library

Library of Congress Cataloging-in-Publication Data available

Hospital Infection Control
for Nurses

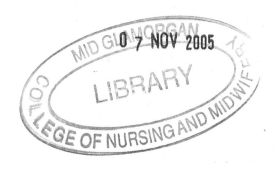

Contents

Preface

'How-to-do-it' books differ. Some give precise instructions, others describe the tools, and readers are left to use them according to circumstances. Conditions in hospitals vary enormously, and so we have followed the latter pattern. Basic information on infection control is provided to allow rational, cost-effective choices to be made, tailored to local need and resources. We hope it will be useful to health professionals working in countries at all levels of socioeconomic development and in any type of health-care system.

To meet this specification, we have examined the roots of current practice. If we find these wanting, we say so. This is not simple anarchy. The average individual can no longer afford lifetime medical care to modern standards. Attempts to make this a collective responsibility through insurance or taxation have not succeeded. The result is rationing. In richer countries, this operates either by putting the full range of medical care out of the reach of less affluent citizens, or elsewhere by making them wait months or years for treatment. Poorer countries see the cost of services they would like to introduce rise faster than their national incomes. In these circumstances, anything that can reduce the cost of medical care without affecting its quality must be welcome. Of course, we have not found a solution to a problem that has eluded others. We claim only to add savings that may be derived from a critical appraisal of current practices to the significant benefits already available from the application of effective infection control policies.

In assembling our material we have tried to be brief yet comprehensive. There are numerous textbooks on microbiology and infectious diseases. We include here only as much of these subjects as are particularly relevant, or necessary for immediate comprehension. We have delved a little into history. We believe this is important, particularly in cases where current practice reflects past errors or misconceptions.

The book is intended for medical and nursing practitioners in infection control and nurse educators. We think much of it might be read with benefit by hospital administrators, medical students, those concerned with the central supply of diagnostic and therapeutic materials and, indeed, anyone whose duties involve direct or indirect contact with patients.

Peter Meers
Wendy Jacobsen
Madeleine McPherson

Abbreviations

AIDS	Acquired immune deficiency syndrome, due to infection with the HIV
APIC	Association of Practitioners of Infection Control
CAI	Community acquired infection
CDC	Centers for Disease Control, 1600 Clifton Road, N.E. Atlanta, GA, 30333, USA
CFC	Chlorofluorocarbon
CIO	Control of infection officer
CSSD	Central sterile supply department
EO	Ethylene oxide
GI	Gastrointestinal infection
GNR	Gram-negative, rod-shaped bacteria
HAI	Hospital acquired (nosocomial) infection
HCW	Health care worker
HEPA	High-efficiency particulate air (filtration)
HIV	Human immunodeficiency virus (see AIDS)
HSDU	Hospital sterilization and disinfection unit
ICC	Infection control committee
ICI	Intravascular cannula-associated infection
ICN	Infection control nurse
ICNA	Infection Control Nurses' Association
ICT	Infection control team
ICU	Intensive care unit
LRI	Lower respiratory infection
MARSA	Methicillin and aminoglycoside resistant *Staphylococcus aureus*
MRC	Medical Research Council (UK)
MRSA	Methicillin-resistant *Staphylococcus aureus*
NUH	National University Hospital, Kent Ridge, Singapore 0511
OR	Operating room
OD	Operating department
PML	Polymorphonuclear leucocyte

RTI	Respiratory tract infection
SENIC	Study on the efficacy of nosocomial infection control
SWI	Surgical wound infection
TPN	Total parenteral nutrition
TSSU	Theatre sterile supply unit
UTI	Urinary tract infection
uV	Ultraviolet (light)

Part One

Infection in hospitals

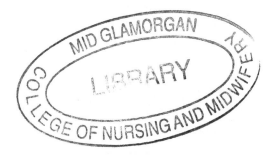

Chapter 1

History

THE BACKGROUND

Infection is a painful fact of life and the chief cause of death. Even where major infectious killers have nearly disappeared and diseases of old age are common, in the end it is often infection that turns debility into mortality. It is no surprise that a fear of infection is deeply rooted in the human consciousness.

In very early times, disease was regarded as a supernatural punishment for sin. When ancient philosophers discarded this idea and began to separate infectious from non-infectious diseases, they developed two opinions of how infections spread. Some argued it was by contact between individuals directly, or indirectly by way of inanimate objects passed between them. This was called contagion, and a logical development of the theory required there to be some kind of particle that was 'infectious'. Others believed infection was the result of inhaling toxic emanations from the earth. These 'miasmas' were often accompanied by smells, so the foul odour of putrefaction was dangerous. To prevent contagion, those afflicted were isolated. In the case of leprosy this was for life, otherwise it might be for 40 days, as the name quarantine suggests. Miasma was avoided by flight from the source of toxic emanations, or it was removed by clearing away the sources of smells. In the absence of experimental observation, illogical arguments between miasmatists and contagionists continued until the middle of the nineteenth century.

In the eighteenth century the contagious nature of gonorrhoea was self-evident to Samuel Johnson's rather promiscuous biographer James Boswell, but how cholera, typhoid and tuberculosis were spread by contact was not clear. Until the part played by blood-sucking insects and other arthropods had been discovered, miasma was as good an explanation as any for the otherwise unaccountable transmission of malaria, plague or yellow fever. The argument lingers to this day in the doubts some people have about the relative importance of personal (contagious) and environmental (miasmic) factors as the cause of infections in hospitals.

In ancient times, hospitals were places to which slaves and later the poor and homeless were sent when they were ill, injured or insane. Their prime function was to keep the sick out of sight rather than to cure them. Although this tradition was gradually overlaid by more humanitarian developments, traces of it persisted well into this century. Until very recently, those who could afford it were treated at home. In the Middle Ages, typhus and relapsing fever spread death equally in hospital ward and prison cell. In the middle of the nineteenth century, Simpson (1869) recorded that nearly a quarter of 7264 amputees had died after surgery in the preceding decade in England, Scotland and Wales. In 1856, the overall death-rate following childbirth in the Paris *Maternite* is said to have been 6%. Most of these deaths were caused by infections.

It is usual (though not necessarily accurate) to date the first scientific attempt to control infections in hospitals to 1844 (Semmelweiss, 1861). In that year, the Hungarian Ignaz Semmelweis was appointed to the Obstetric Division of the Vienna General Hospital. This had two clinics: medical students were taught in the first, and midwives were trained in the second. It was common knowledge that the death-rate was higher in the first clinic. Semmelweis set out to investigate this, and he began what is now regarded as a classical study by measuring the size of the difference. Although it varied from time to time, in the six years 1840–6 he found the average mortality had been 10% in the first clinic, and 3% in the second. Most deaths were due to puerperal fever, an infection that originated in the wound left when the placenta separated. Semmelweis looked for its cause and for a way to prevent it. In his search he was helped by the existence of the two clinics. One after another he altered methods and practices in the first clinic, and waited to see if this had any effect on the mortality there, compared with the second. Semmelweis may have been the first epidemiologist to use 'test' and 'control' groups in this way. Also, by making changes one at a time, he avoided confusing their effects.

Semmelweis found the cause of the excess mortality and discovered how to reduce it, though the experiment took a long time and cost many lives. Bacteriological insight would have made the task easier, but this did not become available for another 30 or 40 years. Medical students were taught the elements of obstetrics on the bodies of women who had died after childbirth, many of puerperal fever. Staff and students moved freely from post-mortem room to bedside. By 1847 Semmelweis had deduced that a contagious substance was spread from the dead to the living on the hands of staff. His control group of midwives were instructed using models, and did not visit the post-mortem room. He made staff and students in the first clinic wash their hands with a disinfectant after leaving the post-mortem room, before tending their patients. The mortality in the first clinic immediately fell to match that in the second. When he introduced handwashing between examining successive patients, the mortality fell to less than 1% in the whole of the obstetrics division.

Unfortunately, Semmelweis was a poor communicator. When his ideas were challenged, he called his colleagues murderers and antagonized everyone to the extent that he was forced to leave. His work and results were ignored and it took another century to rediscover the importance of hands in the transmission of infection in hospitals. A second important deduction might have been made from Semmelweis' work. It is certain he was dealing with classical puerperal fever due to *Streptococcus pyogenes*. The walls, floors, bedding, furniture and the air in his clinics must have been extremely heavily contaminated with streptococci, yet handwashing on its own had a dramatic effect. The conclusion ought to have been that the environment, including the air, could at most have been responsible for only a part of the residual 1% mortality. Semmelweis' unfortunate personality ensured that this strong argument in favour of the theory of contagion fell into obscurity with the rest of his discoveries.

During the early part of the nineteenth century, many of the great cities of the world were equipped with efficient sewers for the first time since the Roman era, and they began to receive supplies of clean water. As open drains and cesspits vanished so did smells, and the separation of sewage and water led to a marked reduction in the incidence of enteric diseases. These simultaneous changes were linked as cause and effect, so strengthening the position of the miasmatists.

Paradoxically, the birth of the science of microbiology further encouraged the miasmatists' belief that infection is spread through the air. Louis Pasteur's interest in fermentation led him into a dispute with those who believed in the spontaneous generation of life. Pasteur showed that living things appeared in nutrient fluids only if they were exposed to the air, so that small airborne particles could fall into them. By 1864 his experiments had disposed of the theory of spontaneous generation, and at the same time they proved that air contains the 'germs' of putrefaction. The fact that these were present in small numbers, and were not generally of the kinds that cause human disease did not emerge until much later. The experiment was impressive, and easily repeated. The surgeon Joseph Lister did so and concluded: '. . . putrefaction in surgical practice is due to particles of dust ever present in the atmosphere'. For him putrefaction was synonymous with infection. He attacked the particles of dust in the operating room with his famous carbolic spray, and because John Tyndall had shown that cotton wool could filter particles out of the air, he used this as a dressing to protect wounds postoperatively. Lister began to practice antiseptic surgery in 1867, and immediately achieved an impressive reduction in post-surgical infection (Lister, 1871). In fact, his success had more to do with the disinfectant action of the spray that settled on otherwise unsterile hands, instruments and, perhaps, particularly on ligatures and sutures, rather than to an effect on the air. Lister eventually realized this, and renounced his earlier belief at the Tenth International Medical Congress in Berlin: '. . . I feel ashamed that I should have ever recommended it' (Lister, 1890). By then 'aseptic' surgery had almost completely replaced the antiseptic variety.

It was some time before the principal implications of the new science of microbiology were accepted. Florence Nightingale believed passionately that disease in general could be banished by cleanliness and fresh air, and she rejected the idea that germs might cause infections. In 1871 the press of the time praised the style used for building the new St Thomas's hospital on the south bank of the Thames in London for not congregating too many patients under one roof for '. . . it is now well known that . . . walls, ceilings and floors become saturated with mephitic odours . . . (that) give rise to those terrible after-consequences of operations known as hospital gangrene'.

A feature of microbiology that is simultaneously a strength and a weakness is an ability to detect biological material in minute quantities. For most of the time since the science was founded over 100 years ago, microbiologists have routinely used methods of much greater sensitivity than were available to other scientists. The weakness of this is that numbers of microbes many times fewer than are required to cause infections are easily detected in the laboratory. For a long time, the enthusiastic pursuit of microbes of no relevance to infection caused much inappropriate activity.

Although the streptococcus was not described until 1877, it was quickly identified as an important pathogen, and recognized as a cause of the most serious kinds of infection in hospitals. By the turn of the century, the situation had improved since the days of Semmelweis, but the death-rate from puerperal sepsis in the 1920s was still two for each 1000 births. Nothing much was done about this until bacteriologists perfected a way to distinguish between different types of *Strep. pyogenes*. This was achieved in the 1930s, and further epidemiological progress was then possible. The new typing scheme showed that streptococcal infections usually arose from patients' attendants and not from patients themselves. This was what Semmelweis had discovered 90 years earlier. It was also found that the environment in the neighbourhood of people carrying streptococci was plentifully contaminated with them. This led to the belief that the environment is an important source of infection.

These findings supplied an apparently scientific basis for the introduction of a number of control measures. These included the isolation of infected or carrier patients, the regular swabbing of staff to locate carriers, who were excluded from work until cleared, the practice of damp dusting, sterilization of bedding, the use of filtered air in special environments like operating rooms, the increased use of disinfectants and antiseptics, and so on (Williams *et al.*, 1966). These measures were introduced in a blunderbuss fashion so their individual effectiveness was not measured. It is likely that Semmelweis would have been puzzled by the need for some of them, and he is certain to have disapproved of the lack of controlled studies to show they worked. The introduction of sulphonamides in 1936, and penicillin a little later further confused the picture. By 1946, the mortality from puerperal fever had fallen to three for each 10 000 births. Much of the credit for this goes to the antimicrobial drugs. Later it was shown that streptococci are damaged by exposure to the air after they are shed from the body. Although they can still be detected by growing them in the laboratory, other than in special circumstances they can no longer cause infections (Chapter 2, p. 35).

Right at the end of the streptococcal era there was an important development in the treatment of surgical wounds. In the 1930s and 1940s, war injuries were a major problem, and the technique of delayed primary suture was very properly reintroduced to prevent gas gangrene. This converts a wound into something resembling a third-degree burn, with the same outstanding potential for colonization and infection. In one series, the incidence of streptococcal colonizations or infections rose from 8% at operation to 30% 14 days later, while those due to staphylococci doubled from a starting point of about 40% (Miles, 1944). The deduction was obvious: wounds were being infected postoperatively, in the ward. The result was the introduction of the 'no touch' dressing technique. Both the idea and the technique have persisted. As most peacetime surgical wounds are closed immediately and become impervious to microbial invasion from the outside after a few hours, this is illogical.

When the streptococcus disappeared as the principal hospital pathogen in the mid-1940s, it was replaced by the staphylococcus. Although infections due to it had always been more common, the lower virulence of staphylococci explains why they were ignored while the more pathogenic streptococci were prevalent. Once *Staphylococcus aureus* had been unmasked by the disappearance of streptococci, it consolidated its position by becoming resistant to penicillin. This it achieved by producing an enzyme (penicillinase or beta-lactamase) that destroys the drug. Staphylococci were perceived as the most important causes of infections in hospitals until 1960 when methicillin, the first of a series of penicillins resistant to penicillinase, was introduced. The Gram-positive cocci were replaced by a succession of Gram-negative, rod-shaped bacteria (GNRs). These caused outbreaks of infection that were noticed because nothing else was happening. They were also more difficult to treat because the GNRs responsible had become resistant to many of the broad-spectrum antimicrobial drugs available at the time. Although they still were (and are) a problem, they were pushed back into relative obscurity in 1976 by the reappearance of the staphylococcus, in a new form. It was now resistant to methicillin (so to all penicillins and cephalosporins) and to the aminoglycoside antimicrobial, gentamicin. At the time of writing, infections with methicillin and aminoglycoside resistant *Staph. aureus* (MARSA) are attracting a lot of attention in hospitals in many parts of the world.

REFERENCES

Lister, J. (1871) The address in surgery. *Brit. Med. J.*, **2**, 225–33.

Lister, J. (1890) The present position of antiseptic surgery. *Brit. Med. J.*, **2**, 377–9.

Miles, A. A. (1944) Epidemiology of wound infections. *Lancet*, **ii**, 809–14.

Semmelweis, I. P. (1861) *Die Aetiologie, der Begriff, und die Prophylaxis des Kindbettfiebers*. Pest, Wein u. Leipzig.

Simpson, J. Y. (1869) Some comparisons, etc. between limb amputations in the country practices and in the practices of large metropolitan hospitals. *Edinburgh Med. J.*, **15**, 523–32.

Williams, R. E. O., Blowers, R., Garrod, L. P. *et al.* (1966) *Hospital Infection* 2nd edn, Lloyd-Luke, London, pp. 9–21.

Chapter 2

Basic Facts

COLONIZATION AND INFECTION

Colonizations and infections are caused by microbes, that is by viruses, bacteria, algae, protozoa, fungi or by members of a group of very small infectious agents that have been called viroids or prions. These differ from each other and from animals and plants in ways described in microbiology books. Viruses excepted, microbes possess all the characteristics of living creatures. Viruses are very small with space for little more than the instructions they need to duplicate themselves. A mature virus particle is not really alive. Its potential for life is fulfilled when it enters and multiplies inside a cell of some other living thing. Microbes are by far the most numerous life-forms on earth. Most are beneficial, and animals, plants and the human race itself could not exist without them. A few attack creatures to cause infections. Larger parasites, such as worms, are not microbes and the diseases they cause are infestations rather than infections.

From shortly after birth to beyond the grave, every human being is host to enormous numbers of microbes. Among these microbes bacteria cause most of the infections that develop in hospitals, so they attract most attention. Viruses and fungi are next in importance. Bacteria inhabit some of the surfaces of the body, forming a **normal flora**. Each of us carry about 10^{15} of them, or more than 100 000 times more bacteria than there are people on earth. This is why they are so important in hospitals, and why an infection is often caused by bacteria that were already present on the patient before it developed.

From the viewpoint of a bacterium, the human body is divided into two parts. These are depicted in Figure 2.1. The surfaces of the body that are normally inhabited by bacteria make up the first zone, the outer ring. Together these are the **colonized surfaces** of the body. In healthy people, the inside of the circle is kept free of microbes, and so forms the **forbidden zone**. This has two parts, the **privileged surfaces**, usually free of bacteria, and the normally sterile **internal tissues** of the

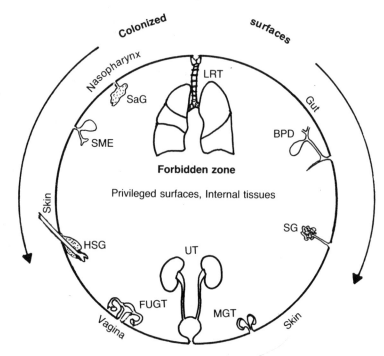

Figure 2.1 A 'bacteria-eye view' of the human body. The colonized surfaces (skin, gastrointestinal tract, etc.) are on the outside, and the 'forbidden zone' kept free of microbes in health, is in the centre. The forbidden zone is subdivided into the 'privileged surfaces' that are structurally continuous with the colonized surfaces (the lower respiratory and urinary tracts, etc.) and the internal tissues (solid organs, cardiovascular system, etc.). Key: LRT, lower respiratory tract; BPD, bile and pancreatic ducts: SG, sweat gland and the breast, MGT, FUGT, male, and female upper genital tracts; UT urinary tract; HSG, hair and sebaceous gland; SME, sinuses and middle ear; SaG, salivary gland.

body. Much of what is conventionally thought of as 'inside' the body is really a part of its surface. The lungs, gastrointestinal and genitourinary tracts, for example, could not perform their biological functions if they were shut off from the outside world. The privileged surfaces that are folded away out of sight have an area many times greater than the visible skin. It is important to recognize this because most of the infections that develop in hospitals begin when microbes normally present on a colonized surface spread to invade a privileged one.

The outcome of a meeting between microbes and a new host depends on three things. These are the relative strengths of the individual's resistance (**host resistance**, the degree to which his or her defence mechanisms are effective); the **virulence** of the attacking microbe (the level of its pathogenicity); and the **number of invaders** (the size of the challenge dose). All three factors vary widely, so in any given case the result is difficult to predict. Microbes that make a challenge usually fail to gain a foothold. Sometimes they succeed and establish themselves and begin to multiply on the surface of the host. If the host does not react, the microbe is regarded as a **non-pathogen** and becomes a **commensal** as a new part of the host's normal flora. If the host reacts in an observable way, an infection is established and the microbe is a **pathogen**. An individual with an infection may become ill (suffer from a **clinical infection**) or the reaction may be so mild that it can only be detected by laboratory tests (a **subclinical** or **asymptomatic infection**). In either case, the body is reacting to some change in the distribution of microbes on it or in it.

Infections are unique among diseases because they involve two distinct living systems. To understand infections, it is necessary to know something about each of the parties, and how they interact. On the human side there is considerable variation in the vigour of an individual's response to microbial attack. The normal human body has a remarkable array of defences against microbes. This **immune system** is incompletely developed in the very young, or it may be permanently defective due to an in-born error. It is temporarily weakened in pregnancy and parts of it wear out as we get older. It is disturbed by illness (particularly malignant disease), and medical or surgical treatment may inactivate or bypass parts of it. Any or all of these causes of immune deficiency lower individuals' resistance to infection to cause **immunocompromise** when it is temporary or **immunodeficiency** when permanent. The result of a deliberate attack on immunity is **immunosuppression**.

Body defences are of two kinds. The first is permanent and present from birth, or develops soon after. This **innate** immune system is made up of non-specific physical, chemical and cellular barriers that act unselectively against most microbes. Second is an **adaptive** immune system. This responds to an infection by producing defences (of which antibodies are an example) that are selectively tailored to the microbe responsible. These act to terminate the infection and then persist to prevent another attack by the same microbe. The innate system provides the principal barrier to what otherwise would be an inevitable invasion of privileged surfaces by microbes from contiguous colonized ones (Figure 2.1). A feature of hospital treatment is the frequency with which such things as surgical wounds, urinary catheters and endotracheal tubes bypass these defensive barriers. The bypasses allow microbes to penetrate the forbidden zone to cause colonizations and infections in places otherwise inaccessible to them. Infections that arise as a direct consequence of these or other forms of treatment are called **iatrogenic**.

On the microbial side, a complete spectrum exists between commensals and pathogens, representing every possible degree of virulence. Those that occupy the intermediate part of the range are **potential** or **opportunistic pathogens**. Fully virulent pathogens may cause infections in healthy people. To do so they must be introduced in sufficient numbers by the correct route, and the individual must not be immune already due to a previous infection with the same pathogen, or as the result of vaccination. An example is the measles virus which nearly always causes disease when first met with in its wild (natural) form. If the first meeting is with the heavily modified virus used in measles vaccine, the result is an asymptomatic infection. In either case, immunity prevents further attack by the virus. The situation is entirely different in patients suffering from an immune deficiency. Such patients can be infected by microbes of low virulence invading in small numbers. Because patients do not respond properly, repeated attacks are possible. Depending on the severity of the deficiency, infections may be caused by opportunistic pathogens and even commensals. In extreme circumstances, the line that divides pathogens from non-pathogens disappears.

The other important variable is the size of the challenge dose. The defences of the body can repel surprisingly large numbers of bacteria. For instance, one million *Staph. aureus* must be injected into healthy skin to produce a small pustule. Ten million painted on to intact skin are without effect. The situation is different if immunity is compromised. One hundred *Staph. aureus* on a suture will produce a stitch abscess. The presence of this small foreign body is sufficient to reduce immune competence by a factor of 10 000 (Elek and Conen, 1957).

The normal flora of the body is complex, with a powerful built-in resistance to change. Bacteria from the environment that attempt to take up residence rarely succeed. This resistance to colonization depends on the existence of a balanced normal flora. If the balance is upset, some existing components may overgrow, or new colonists establish themselves much more easily. Treatment with antimicrobial drugs, exposure to antiseptics and a change of diet (all common in hospitals) tend to upset the balance. This is why most patients add to their normal flora some new colonists soon after they are admitted to hospital. These newcomers are acclimatized to life in hospital. They are more resistant to antimicrobial drugs and more easily take advantage of the special circumstances of patient care. In general, these 'hospital bacteria' do not threaten healthy, immunocompetent people, and so do not often cause infections among hospital staff. For the same reason, patients who leave hospital carrying some of them are not a threat to their friends and relatives. When patients regain health and immune competence, any hospital bacteria they still carry tend to be replaced by a healthy normal flora.

The surface of the human body resembles many other biological systems in which a mixture of different living things come to terms with each other and achieve an ecological balance. Such systems have several things in common. For example, in a 'healthy' primary jungle, a large number of different species of trees, plants, animals, birds, insects and so on live together in a balanced state, with each species present in relatively small numbers. If the primary jungle is destroyed, it is replaced by an 'unhealthy' secondary jungle. This contains many fewer different species, but with each of them present in larger numbers. For example, rodents may proliferate in a secondary jungle. These may carry microbes hazardous to humans, and therefore diseases such as leptospirosis, scrub typhus and plague become more common.

There are similarities in the ecological sense between a secondary jungle and what happens in hospitals. In the healthy state, the surface of the human body carries many different microbial species that live together in a balanced state. In an unhealthy unbalanced state, as in a secondary jungle, a smaller number of species is found with one or more of them present in abnormally large numbers. The major difference between a primary rain forest and the surface of the human body is that in the jungle the life-span of many of the species is measured in years or decades. On the body, microbial life-spans are measured in minutes. In a few hours, a healthy normal flora can become an unhealthy one. Fortunately, the opposite is also true, and 'health' is regained in a few days rather than the centuries it takes to remake a primary jungle.

Infections are inseparable from communal life, but they are more common and more severe in hospitals than elsewhere. Some patients come into hospital for the treatment of established infections, and others are more or less debilitated by the illnesses for which they are admitted. Treatment commonly causes further debility. A vicious circle is created in which patients with infections are mixed with those more likely to acquire them, and fuel is added as more susceptible patients are admitted to replace those who are discharged or die. The control of infection in hospitals has been likened to digging a well and then trying to keep the water out! Infections that develop are treated with antimicrobial drugs. The scale of the problem is such that at any one time at least 20% of patients in hospitals are receiving these drugs. They may be given for the treatment of established or imagined infections, or as prophylactics to try to prevent them. Bacteria that survive in this environment are selected because they can resist the antimicrobials in use. This is how 'hospital strains' of bacteria emerge to grow vigorously in the fertile seed-bed provided for them.

Modern medical or surgical treatments almost inevitably cause some reduction in host resistance to infection. For a patient whose defences are doubly weakened by his or her illness and the effects of treatment, a commensal becomes an opportunistic pathogen, and an opportunistic pathogen a full pathogen. This deterioration in host resistance is responsible for most infections that develop in hospitals. The microbes that cause the infections are often ones that patients brought into hospital with them, or that were added to their 'normal' flora after admission. Patients with severe immune deficiency may develop septicaemias secondarily to quite minor tissue infections. These arise from small accidental or therapeutic breaks in the epithelial surfaces of the skin, gut, respiratory or urinary tracts caused by intravascular or urethral catheterization, endoscopy and so on. The bacteria that take advantage of these defects vary according to the flora (normal or disordered) of the site involved. Such patients have often been in hospital for some time, so they are likely to be colonized by less desirable, multi-resistant hospital strains of bacteria. This is the situation in intensive care units, where patients disadvantaged by severe disability are also more likely to harbour hospital strains among the flora of their colonized surfaces. When an infection develops, there is a good chance that one of these hospital strains will be responsible.

It is clear that some infections are inescapable consequences of admission to hospital. However, there is good evidence that there are more of these infections than need be (Chapter 3, p. 47), though the irreducible minimum has not been defined. It may never be, because the target is moving. As medical science develops, ever more debilitated patients are subjected to increasingly complex invasive treatments. Although these may improve the quality of life for some, the penalty for others is an increase in morbidity and mortality due to infections.

A real practical difficulty arises in making a distinction between an infection and a colonization. This arises when potentially pathogenic bacteria are found as the result of a culture, but it is uncertain if they are there as non-pathogenic commensals (a colonization), or as infecting pathogens.

The difficulty is compounded because a colonization nearly always precedes an infection, perhaps by several days. In the case of classical infections – measles or chicken-pox, for example – the incubation period between microbial entry into the body and the appearance of disease is the time taken to convert the initial colonization into an infection. In these cases, the change from one state to the other is abrupt and obvious. In other cases, and particularly with infections in hospitals, the point at which a colonization becomes an infection (if indeed it ever does) may be difficult or impossible to determine.

An example of this difficulty is the case of a pressure sore (bedsore or decubitus ulcer). Destruction of skin leads to exposure of subcutaneous tissues and the establishment of a moist area rich in bacterial nutrients, but with a poor blood supply that limits the body's capacity to react. Different kinds of bacteria take advantage of this, and various staphylococci, streptococci and, for instance, *Pseudomonas aeruginosa* may be found on the surface of the ulcer. More often than not, the presence of these microbes represents a colonization. A decision to call it an infection requires care, for two reasons. First, this is the point at which antimicrobial drugs are likely to be prescribed. Their use in this situation is unlikely to do anything other than ensure a continued supply of hospital strains of bacteria. Secondly, the patient is then listed among those who have acquired an infection in hospital. The criteria for making the diagnosis of an infection (recognized as particularly difficult to apply in this case) are the presence or absence of the classical signs of inflammation (pain, swelling, redness, heat and loss of function). Other examples of this difficulty will be mentioned later.

When two or more infections are clearly related to each other an **outbreak** or **epidemic** of infection exists, though the latter term is usually reserved for examples involving large numbers of people. When cases of influenza appear in a community, the existence of an epidemic is fairly obvious. In hospitals, the situation is different, and it is necessary to be much more rigorous in determining the identity of the microbes isolated from the patients concerned. To show that there is an outbreak of, say, wound infection requires that the bacteria causing the individual cases are, so far as it is possible to determine, 'the same' (below, p. 26). It is not enough to note only that the infections seem to be related in time and that the patients concerned are connected by the part of the hospital where they were housed, or by the member of staff who treated them.

FREQUENCY AND TYPES OF INFECTION IN HOSPITALS

Infections found in hospitals are of two kinds. Those brought into hospital or being incubated on admission are **community acquired**

infections (CAI), while those that appear in hospital after admission and are due to it are **hospital acquired infections** (HAI). Some use the expression **nosocomial infection** rather than HAI – the terms are synonymous. HAI is simply defined as:

> 'An infection found in a patient in hospital that was not present and was not being incubated on admission, or having been acquired in hospital, appeared after discharge.'

If desired, this definition can be extended to include infections of members of hospital staff that result from their employment.

It is nearly always very easy to distinguish between CAI and HAI. Difficult cases are usually resolved by careful examination of records or the patient. Other than after prosthetic surgery, it is rarely necessary to use an arbitrary distinction based on the time of appearance of an infection in relation to hospital admission. As a last resort, an infection that appears before the third day in hospital may be labelled CAI, and after that, HAI.

A more serious and frequent difficulty arises in trying to distinguish between a colonization and an infection (above, p. 14). If doubt persists after all available information has been taken into account, it may be necessary to defer judgement until the situation clarifies in the following days. This problem is referred to again when the different infections are discussed (Chapter 4).

When it has been measured in more developed countries, the prevalence of CAI in a hospital has approximately equalled that of HAI present at the same time. The kinds of infections that make up CAI vary substantially with the geographical location and degree of development of the community concerned. The composition of HAI is more constant, particularly in developed countries. Of course, allowance must be made for the types of patients being surveyed. A hospital with a heavy surgical load will record more surgical wound infections

Table 2.1 Rates of hospital acquired infections detected by some recent surveys

	Prevalence surveys					Incidence survey	
	Canada	Hong Kong	Scandinavia			UK	USA
HAI rate %	8.2	8.9	10.5 10.5 12.1		9.0	9.2	5.7

Note: in the surveys, broadly similar criteria were used and no obvious confounding factors were present. The difference between incidence and prevalence rates is methodological, not real (below p. 38). For dates and references see Table 2.2.

Table 2.2 Hospital acquired infections according to their site as reported from various countries

Infection	Percent of all hospital acquired infections											
	Canada	Hong Kong	Italy	Scandinavia				Singapore	UK	USA		
UTI	39	33	31	42	38	45	42	41	30	36	40	42
SWI	24	24	13	26	18	21	17	26	19	25	24	24
LRI	26	21	18	10	22	12	14	13	16	15	19	11
Other	11	22	28	22	22	22	27	20	35	23	17	23
Date of Survey date	1976	1987	1986	1978	1980	1980	1981	1990	1981	1964	1971	1986

Key: UTI, urinary tract infections; SWI, surgical wound infections; LRI, lower respiratory infections; Other, infections at other sites.

Note: the dates refer to the year of publication of the paper giving the details: Bernander *et al.*, 1978; French *et al.*, 1987; Haley, R. W., 1986; Hinton, 1976; Hovig *et al.*, 1981; Jepsen and Mortensen, 1980; Kislak *et al.*, 1964; Meers *et al.*, 1981; Meers and Leong, 1990; Moro *et al.*, 1986; Scheckler *et al.*, 1971.

than one where most patients are admitted with medical conditions. Discrepancies also arise because of differences in the average length of time patients spend in hospital. This varies from place to place, and seems to be falling everywhere. Although infections that appear after discharge should be included in the count of cases of HAI, this is difficult to achieve. The result is that infections that may take time to become evident, for example, surgical infections, are increasingly under-represented as the hospital stay shortens. Despite these factors, similarities outweigh differences in the amounts and types of HAI found in acute hospitals in countries with different systems of health care. This is illustrated in Tables 2.1 and 2.2.

In each of the surveys, urinary tract infections (UTI) were the most common, causing between 30% and 45% of cases of HAI. Surgical wound infections (SWI, 13–26% of HAI) were the next most common in eight surveys, while lower respiratory infections (LRI, 10–26% of HAI) came second in four. Other infections were made up of a number of less frequent causes of HAI. These ranged from infections of the skin (including those of intravascular sites), to the most life-threatening variety, septicaemia. In more developed countries, another of the 'other' infections, gastroenteritis, is a rare cause of HAI in acute hospitals, but in some places it is frequent, particularly among children. It is everywhere more common among long-stay patients, especially if they need psychiatric care. It is caused by inadequate communal and personal hygiene.

A feature of the results of surveys in which cases of HAI are counted is that they usually record more infections than infected patients, and more microbial causes of infection than infections. The reason is that a patient with one HAI, say of the urinary tract, is at increased risk of developing septicaemia and perhaps pneumonia as well if the causative microbe spreads into the blood. Thus one patient may suffer from two or three different HAIs, and these are counted as separate episodes. Also, a single infection is sometimes caused by two or more microbes acting together. For example, pus from a surgical wound may contain aerobic and anaerobic bacteria, with both contributing to the pathology.

DISTRIBUTION OF INFECTIONS

The infections described in the last section are not distributed evenly throughout a hospital. Patients in some departments or units suffer from HAI more frequently than others, and the different kinds of infection are also spread unevenly. The distribution of infections is

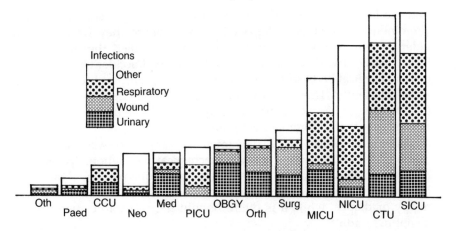

Figure 2.2 The amounts and types of hospital acquired infections found in different units and departments in the National University Hospital, Singapore, in the four years 1986–9. The heights of the columns are directly proportional to the incidence of infection in each unit.

Key: Oth, other departments; Paed, paediatric department; CCU, coronary care unit; Neo, neonatal unit; Med, general medicine; PICU, paediatric intensive care unit; OBGY, obstetrics and gynaecology; Orth, orthopaedic department; Surg, general surgery; MICU, medical intensive care unit; NICU, neonatal intensive care unit; CTU, cardiothoracic unit; SICU, surgical intensive care unit.

illustrated here using information collected over a four-year period in the National University Hospital (NUH), Singapore (Meers and Leong, 1990). During this time, HAI was surveyed by means of a partial incidence study, the mechanism of which is described in Chapter 3 (p. 52).

Figure 2.2 shows where HAI was found in NUH, and the distribution of its types, by speciality. The greatest weight of infection fell on four of the six intensive care units. Patients in the worst-affected areas suffered from HAI more than 16 times as often as those in the least affected, who occupied beds allocated to the ophthalmic, ear, nose and throat and dental surgery departments. Because the survey was only partial, absolute numbers of infections are not given, but the incidences shown by the heights of the columns in Figure 2.2 are proportional to each other. The general distribution found agrees with that in other advanced countries (Table 2.2).

The comparatively heavy concentration of UTI among obstetric and gynaecological patients is notable. This is a consequence of the anatomical location of the procedures carried out in this department, and the large use made of catheters. Catheters also accounted for the prominence of UTI in orthopaedic wards, where they were used in older patients confined to bed. There they equalled the numbers of SWIs, many of which were associated with road accidents. Patients in general surgical beds suffered from UTIs less often, but LRIs appeared more frequently. This was a result of the general effect of anaesthesia (Chapter 4, p. 76) sometimes complicated by reduced respiratory movement after abdominal operations.

The concentration of LRIs in intensive care units was due to the number of patients who required mechanical ventilation. In the two paediatric intensive care units, UTIs were uncommon. This may be because no one worries too much if a infant or child has a wet nappy or diaper, while it is often thought necessary to catheterize an incontinent adult.

MICROBIAL CAUSES OF INFECTIONS

The microbes least likely to cause any kind of infection are the algae. Algae, like plants, normally need light to grow, so cannot easily invade tissues or cause trouble under clothing or dressings. However, recent experience has shown that some algae produce very toxic products. There have been incidents in which people and animals have been poisoned as a result of exposure to them. For this reason, algae should not be dismissed out of hand as possible pathogens in human infections. Fungi cause infections of two kinds. Those found in surface infections, such as ringworm or athlete's foot, can only grow in the horny layer of the skin, or in the hair and nails. They (and the algae) rarely invade deeper tissues. Other fungi, most commonly *Candida albicans*, are able to cause deep infections. *C. albicans* is of low virulence, so although it may cause superficial infections in apparently healthy people, it only invades the tissues of those whose immunity is severely impaired. The number of patients in this cateogry grows year by year as more enterprising techniques are used to treat malignant diseases or repair or replace damaged organs, and as the pandemic of human immunodeficiency virus (HIV) infection and the acquired immune deficiency syndrome (AIDS) spreads. Some others of the less pathogenic fungi appear as pathogens in severely immunodeficient patients. Among these, *Aspergillus* spp. or *Pneumocystis carinii* also cause serious infections. The classification of the latter opportunistic pathogen, for long regarded as a protozoon, is in doubt. Recent work suggests that it more closely resembles a fungus (Edman *et al.*, 1988).

Some respiratory viruses and enteroviruses may cause sharp outbreaks of HAI among groups of susceptible patients. Viral respiratory tract infections, gastroenteritis or meningitis can be troublesome in infants, and influenza is a significant cause of morbidity and mortality in geriatric units. However, viruses are not a special threat to the mass of acute hospital patients, so are not conspicuous causes of HAI. Again, patients with impaired immunity form a special group who are likely to be attacked by members of the herpes group of viruses. These cause primary infections in the same way as other viruses, but unlike what follows in most cases, they do not disappear afterwards. Instead, they establish themselves permanently in a proportion of the cells they infect. Here they hide away without (at least initially) causing any harm. This property is called **latency**.

Latent viruses may be reactivated later to cause recurrent infections. Sufferers from cold sores due to the herpes simplex virus are uncomfortably aware of this tendency. Patients with shingles are experiencing a recurrent infection with another member of the herpes group, the varicella-zoster virus. This was left behind in latent form after an attack of chicken-pox, often in childhood. Reactivation of the virus to cause shingles is more frequent and severe as the efficiency of the immune system is reduced. Elderly people or people being treated for malignancy are often nursed together. Shingles is much more likely to appear among such patients. By chance, two or three cases may coexist giving the false impression that there is an outbreak. It has to be stressed that chicken pox (varicella) and shingles (herpes zoster) are part of the same infection, usually extended over many years. Either is infectious, but only to someone who has not previously had chicken-pox. A non-immune person exposed to chicken-pox or shingles is likely to develop chicken-pox. Exposure to shingles does not cause shingles.

With increasing immunological deficiency, other less pathogenic members of the herpes group (the cytomegalovirus and Epstein-Barr viruses) begin to cause serious disease. This pattern is repeated with a few of the protozoa, and even some of the worms that may infest man. The protozoon *Toxoplasma gondii* is an example. Many people share this parasite with their cats, in most cases without knowing it. This is another latent infection that may be activated and cause serious disease in patients whose immunity is impaired.

Patients who receive transplanted organs or other tissues must be immunosuppressed to prevent rejection of their transplants. Latent microbes may already be present in the recipient. More dangerously they may be transferred in the donated tissue or a blood transfusion to a recipient who has not previously encountered that pathogen. In either case, the immunosuppression necessary to preserve the transplant may also cause reactivation of the latent microbe, with potentially serious consequences.

A new and increasingly common cause of immunodeficiency is HIV. Although this causes a community acquired infection, the end stage, AIDS, usually presents in hospitals. AIDS develops after a period of months or years during which HIV has attacked and destroyed an important part of the immune system. The patient is then subject to repeated attacks of infections due to one or more of the microbes already mentioned, plus some others that can take advantage of immunosuppression. They may also develop certain forms of cancer that are normally suppressed by the immune system. Most of the infections suffered by a patient with AIDS are caused by microbes that are weakly or completely non-pathogenic for normal people, so they do not threaten the staff of hospitals. Tuberculosis is one infection for which this is not true.

Once it has been acquired, an HIV infection seems to develop slowly but relentlessly until its terminal stage, AIDS, is reached. This progression is at best only slowed down by treatment. The possibility that the such an infection may be 'caught' by occupational exposure is a common cause of concern among health care workers. HIV is nearly always acquired through sexual activity with an infected person, or by practices (including intravenous drug abuse with shared syringes) that involve the exchange of significant amounts of body fluids, and blood in particular. It is extremely rare for health care workers (HCWs) to acquire HIV infections as a result of occupational exposure to infected patients. HCWs can protect themselves from the very small risk of infection by taking simple precautions ('universal precautions', Chapter 5, p. 94; and by avoiding 'sharps' injuries, Chapter 5, p. 126). Patients themselves are protected in those countries where donors of tissues or blood used therapeutically are examined to exclude the possibility that they are carrying HIV.

In their more severe forms, all the infections mentioned so far are confined to patients who are severely immunosuppressed. Other than in transplant and oncology units and places where AIDS is common, such patients are unusual, and so in general the number of infections of these kinds is small. Among the very much larger number of patients who do not fall into this category, HAI is commonly due to bacteria. This is because bacteria are already established in large numbers on the body surfaces of patients and members of staff. In consequence, they are poised to take advantage of even small local failures of immunity. Most patients admitted to hospital suffer at least a minor insult to their immune systems, and so are vulnerable.

It is convenient to divide the bacteria that cause HAI into the 'big

Table 2.3 Some characteristics that contribute to the pathogenicity of the major bacterial pathogens in HAI

	Strep. pyogenes	*Staph. aureus*	*Gram-negative rods*
Normal habitat	Pharynx	Nose, moist skin	Gut
Colonization frequency	<5–10%	20–50%	100%
Resistance to drying*	Fair	Good	Nearly all poor
Virulence	High	Moderate	Moderate
Resistance to antimicrobials	Unimportant	Very important	Important
Typical sites of HAI	Skin, wounds, septicaemia	Skin, wounds, septicaemia	Urinary and respiratory tracts, wounds, septicaemia

*But see text.

three' major pathogens, and a miscellaneous group of 'others'. The big three are *Strep. pyogenes* among the streptococci, *Staph. aureus* from the staphylococci (Shanson, 1981; Goldman, 1986), and a number of Gram-negative, rod-shaped bacteria (GNRs), whose similarities in the context of HAI outweigh their differences. The GNRs include *Escherichia coli*, *Klebsiella* spp., *P. aeruginosa*, *Enterobacter*, *Serratia*, *Citrobacter* and *Acinetobacter* spp., plus a few others. The characteristics that make the big three important as causes of HAI are summarized in Table 2.3.

At any one time, medical and nursing staff in hospitals perceive one of the big three pathogens as a greater threat to patients than the others. This pathogen then achieves 'dominance' for the time being, and receives particular attention. In fact, at present, and so far as it can be determined in the past, GNRs have always caused more infections than either of the others put together, and staphylococcal infections have been more common than streptococcal, even when the latter was the 'dominant' cause of HAI.

Historically, the streptococcus has been most feared. Although not identified until the science of bacteriology was founded in the latter half of the nineteenth century, there is no doubt that it was active earlier. The cause of the dominance of the streptococcus is its extreme virulence: it can kill apparently healthy people in a few hours. The other members of the big three do not do this. The introduction of the sulphonamides in the 1930s accelerated what already may have been the beginning of the decline of the streptococcus, and it ceased to be important as a cause of HAI in the 1940s, after the development of penicillin. The virtual disappearance of the streptococcus as a hospital pathogen is usually credited to penicillin, to which it was and is extremely susceptible. However, it is generally agreed that the virulence of the organism had begun to decline prior to the use of antimicrobials. A cyclical waxing and waning of virulence over periods of decades has been postulated for several microbes, including the streptococcus. It would be rash to assume that the streptococcus will not one day return as an important cause of HAI. If this were accompanied by the acquisition of resistance to penicillin, the result would be a problem that would dwarf the current concern about staphylococci.

Work done in the 1930s and 1940s on the epidemiology of hospital infections due to streptococci led to the imposition of a number of infection control measures (Chapter 1, p. 7). One was the practice of screening people bacteriologically for the presence of *Strep. pyogenes*, and excluding from work members of staff or isolating any patients found to be carriers. This was possible due to the low rate of carriage, and so the number of individuals involved was small and disruption was minimal. Many more practices were founded on the discovery that the inanimate environment surrounding patients suffering from streptococcal infections were plentifully contaminated with their streptococci. This gave rise to the idea that bacteriological surveillance of the environment was a useful way of detecting contamination. It also led to the enforcement of a variety of measures, such as damp dusting, the sterilization of bedding, the widespread use of disinfectants, the no-touch technique for dressing wounds, the use of filtered air in operating rooms, and the wearing of masks outside operating departments. None of these was introduced in a controlled fashion, so their effectiveness has never been measured. Although not of proven efficacy, the search for carriers has some logic. However, because the bacteriological examination takes not less than 24 hours to complete, a carrier may already have passed on his or her microbe to another person before being detected. The discovery that streptococci exposed to the air rapidly lose their infectivity (below, p. 35) throws some doubt on the usefulness of environmental measures. Unfortunately, once they had been introduced, they rapidly acquired the force of essential rituals. Most have not been reversed or even critically re-examined, and are still used to protect patients from a risk of unknown size, due to microbes for which they were not designed and against which they were never shown to be effective.

The growing availability of penicillin in the later 1940s was accompanied by an increasing prevalence of staphylococci that had developed resistance to it due to the production of a beta-lactamase (penicillinase). These 'hospital' staphylococci replaced streptococci as the dominant cause of HAI. By 1948, they accounted for 60% of the staphylococci that were isolated in hospitals in the UK; in some places by 1955 the figure had reached 90%. Outbreaks of infection were common. In 1952, a new, more virulent, strain appeared in Australia that was able to cause serious infections in normal people, including members of the staff of hospitals, and even (it was said) to penetrate unbroken skin. This was later called the 80/81 staphylococcus, and it caused alarm as it spread round the world in a pandemic.

In 1960, methicillin, a form of penicillin resistant to beta-lactamase, was introduced. This was active against the hospital staphylococcus, and the 80/81 strain disappeared. Almost immediately, the first strains of methicillin resistant *Staph. aureus* (MRSA) were identified. These spread much more slowly than was the case with the hospital staphylococcus in the 1940s and 1950s, and they were generally regarded as of little importance. In 1976, slightly more pathogenic strains of MRSA that were resistant to the aminoglycoside gentamicin (MARSA) appeared in Australia and the UK. At the time of writing, MARSA has not fully duplicated the ability of the 80/81 pandemic strain to replace other staphylococci, or acquired its virulence. It causes concern because it is necessary to use more expensive and toxic antimicrobial drugs in the treatment of infections due to it. It almost certainly receives more attention and causes more disruption than it warrants.

By contrast, GNRs attract less attention than they deserve. Although almost certainly always the most common causes of HAI, it was only between 1960 and 1976 that GNRs finally achieved the notoriety of dominance. They did this when streptococcal HAI had disappeared and staphylococci were no longer considered a threat. Multiply resistant strains of different GNRs were observed to cause limited outbreaks of HAI in some hospitals (see, for example, Casewell and Phillips, 1978; Chow *et al.*, 1979; Cross *et al.*, 1983; Curie *et al.*, 1978; Pitt *et al.*, 1980). However, when the staphylococcus re-emerged in the form of MARSA, GNRs fell back into comparative obscurity, though of course they did not go away. Figure 2.3 and Table 2.4 show that GNRs still cause most cases of HAI. Proportionately, they cause septicaemia more often than staphylococci. The ability of a microbe to cause septicaemia is often taken as a measure of its pathogenicity. By this criterion, GNRs are no less virulent than staphylococci.

Figure 2.3 and Table 2.4 illustrate the distribution of the major bacterial pathogens by type of infection and speciality, respectively. Because of current interest, distinction is made in the table between methicillin-sensitive *Staph. aureus* and MARSA. The data are from the National University Hospital, Singapore (above, pp. 17 and 18). With

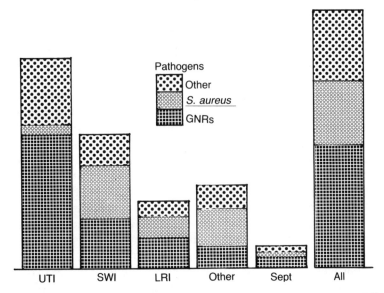

Figure 2.3 The distribution of the major bacterial pathogens causing different HAI in the National University Hospital, Singapore, from January 1986 to December 1989.

Key: UTI, urinary tract infection; SWI, surgical wound infection; LRI, lower respiratory infection; Other, other infections; Sept, septicaemia; All, all infections (drawn to a scale 50% of the others); GNR, Gram-negative, rod-shaped bacteria.

the exception of the high incidence of infections due to MARSA, the relative frequencies of the different pathogens and their distributions agree with similar statistics from other countries.

The principal members of the miscellaneous group of bacterial causes of HAI are streptococci of Group D (mainly *Enterococcus faecalis* and *Strep. bovis*), *Candida* spp. and *Staph. epidermidis*. All were found as common causes of UTI, and numbers of them were isolated from infected wounds and infections of the respiratory tract. *Staph. epidermidis* was also found in infections associated with central vascular lines and the catheters used for peritoneal dialysis. They were also reported as pathogens in some blood cultures.

Because infections due to the major pathogens are so common, if three cases of HAI have been caused by, for instance, *E. coli*, it does not follow that the infections are related to each other. The identification of an outbreak of infection depends on reasonable proof that the three strains of *E. coli* are, as nearly as it is possible to determine, 'the same'. To illustrate this, suppose there have been five cases of

Table 2.4 The distribution of the major bacterial pathogens causing HAI in the National University Hospital, Singapore, from January 1986 to December 1989, according to speciality

| | HAI causative organisms (%) | | | | |
	GNR	ORSA	MARSA	Others	Totals
Surgical intensive care	99 (52)	8 (4)	30 (16)	53 (28)	190
Cardiothoracic unit	46 (48)	9 (9)	18 (19)	22 (23)	95
Neonatal intensive care	39 (20)	29 (15)	66 (33)	65 (33)	199
Medical intensive care	67 (42)	12 (8)	26 (16)	54 (34)	159
General surgery	503 (51)	97 (10)	130 (13)	267 (27)	997
Orthopaedics	236 (52)	39 (9)	90 (20)	85 (19)	450
Obstetrics and gynaecology	391 (46)	122 (14)	7 (1)	323 (38)	843
Paediatric intensive care	8 (28)	4 (14)	9 (31)	8 (28)	29
General medicine	463 (57)	62 (8)	102 (12)	192 (23)	819
Neonatal unit	31 (21)	66 (45)	16 (11)	33 (23)	146
Coronary care	17 (53)	3 (9)	3 (9)	9 (28)	32
Paediatrics	63 (40)	32 (20)	22 (14)	40 (25)	157
Others*	11 (35)	8 (26)	3 (10)	9 (29)	31
Totals	1974 (48)	491 (12)	522 (13)	1160 (28)	4147

*Ophthalmology, ear, nose and throat and oral surgery
Key: GNR, Gram-negative rod-shaped bacteria; ORSA, methicillin sensitive, 'ordinary' *S. aureus*; MARSA, methicillin and aminoglycoside resistant *S. aureus*.

staphylococcal wound infections following operations performed by the same surgical team. On investigation, two members of the team are found to be staphylococcal carriers. Which, if either, might be responsible? As up to 50% of normal people carry *Staph. aureus*, both may be innocent because unless the cases and their bacterial causes are connected there is no outbreak. It is necessary to examine the staphylococci from the five patients and the two members of staff by methods designed to reveal minor differences. If they are all different there is no outbreak. If two or more of them are indistinguishable, the necessary inferences are drawn and precise action can follow. To answer questions like this, various methods have been developed that can reliably determine if two or more strains of most of the important causes of HAI are distinguishable or indistinguishable. Unfortunately, these 'typing schemes' nearly always require scarce or expensive reagents or skills that confine them to reference laboratories. Due to this, urgent decisions may be delayed because of lack of information.

To overcome the problem, microbiology laboratories in hospitals make use of their antimicrobial sensitivity test results. These may allow a preliminary judgement to be made on relatedness, so that a decision can be taken whether or not to proceed with an investigation or take remedial action. If two or more strains have quite different sensitivity patterns, then they are most unlikely to be related and there is little possibility that they come from patients involved in an outbreak of infection. If they are identical, they **may** be the same, and it is sensible to accept that an outbreak might exist. Strains should, of course, be kept for submission to a reference laboratory for final adjudication, if the circumstances warrant it.

SOURCES AND VECTORS OF INFECTIONS

A **source** of infection is the place of origin of an infecting microbe. A **vector** or **vehicle** of infection is the agency or pathway by or through which a microbe is transported to reach a portal of entry on a host. A **portal of entry** is the point on (or in) the host at which the microbe gains a foothold to cause an infection. In natural infections, this may be the respiratory or alimentary tracts, or skin or mucous membrane, or the placenta in infections of a fetus. Diagnostic and therapeutic procedures provide a number of very efficient artificial direct routes for the introduction of microbes to cause iatrogenic infections.

A **reservoir** of infection is a place where an infecting microbe is found. It may also be a source of infection, but only if it is connected to a potential host by a vector. Waste traps of sinks, for example, usually contain large numbers of microbes. In clinical areas, these will include pathogenic bacteria washed from the hands of members of staff. Sink waste traps are reservoirs of pathogenic microbes, but it is difficult to imagine circumstances in which they might be a source of infection. This example can be multiplied many times. Time and money can be saved if reservoirs of microbes (like sink traps) are left alone, unless they are also credible as sources of infection.

When looking for the origin of an infection, it is logical to search for the nearest source (avoiding reservoirs) where microbes indistinguishable from those responsible are present in sufficient numbers to provide an infectious dose. If more than one source is located, it is wise to study first that with the greatest number of microbes. Although biology has a way of ignoring over-simplifications, in many cases the application of this rule will produce a working hypothesis, and lead to the right answer as well.

It is customary and useful to divide the large number of possible sources of infecting microbes into two classes and three categories (Figure 2.4). Following the rule just set out for a patient with an

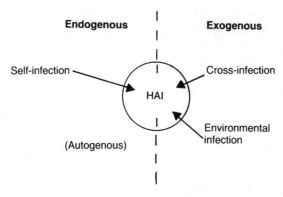

Figure 2.4 Sources of the microbes that cause HAI. Autogenous infections are self-infections with microbes that have colonized the patient following admission to hospital.

infection due to a common organism, the nearest point at which a large number of these are likely to be found is the surface of his or her own body. Infections originating like this are endogenous **self-infections**. As pointed out above (p. 12), patients often acquire new hospital strains of bacteria as members of their 'normal' flora following admission to hospital. If a self-infection with a colonizing hospital strain develops later, the infection is called **autogenous** rather than endogenous. The next most likely source is the surfaces of the bodies of other patients or members of hospital staff. If one of these is the source, the result is an exogenous **cross-infection**. The third possibility is that the infecting microbes came from some part of the environment. These cause exogenous **environmental infections**. It is important to distinguish between self-, cross- and environmental infections, because measures appropriate to the control of HAI differ with the source. Cases of self-infection will not be affected by many of the measures appropriate to environmental infections, so it is a waste of money and effort to apply them.

Self-infection

A self-infection is due to microbes already present on or in the host before the disease process began. In the case of bacterial infections, the source is frequently one of the normally colonized surfaces of the body, though it may be an abnormally colonized privileged surface (above, p. 9) or even an infection at another site. The existence of the latter source ensures that patients suffering from one HAI are more likely to

develop another (above, p. 18). The vector (pathway) may be by direct
spread with extension of the microbe over or through tissues, by
transfer from one part of the body to another on the hands of the
patient or an attendant, or it may be via the blood stream, or through
lymphatics.

The normally colonized surfaces of the body are made up of the
skin, the respiratory tract above the larynx, the gastrointestinal tract
from mouth to anus, and the vagina. The types and numbers of
bacteria that occupy these sites vary enormously. The skin is the
largest organ of the body. It contains hair follicles, sweat and sebaceous
glands, and it includes the nails. It varies in thickness, the extent to
which the surface is cornified, and the degree to which it is moist
(groin, perineum, axillae and flexures) or dry (exposed areas). The
surface is constantly shed at a rate that varies from place to place on
the body, and from person to person. In general, men shed more
than women. Shedding is of flattened, leaf-like squames about 10–20
microns across, which may be shed individually or in groups. When
large numbers adhere together, desquamation is a visible process,
as with dandruff or scaly skin. Significantly more squames are shed
immediately after washing and drying, particularly if powerful detergents are used. Most squames are sterile, but a variable proportion act
as a raft for one or more living bacteria. An average adult loses about
300 million squames a day. If one in a hundred is carrying bacteria, an
individual may shed 2000 of these a minute. In occupied enclosed
spaces, nearly all the bacteria in the air and much of the dust originate
in this way. Minute fibres rubbed from clothing make up a large part of
the rest. Nearly all of these are sterile (Selwyn and Ellis, 1972; Meers
and Yeo, 1978; Noble, 1983).

The normal bacterial flora of the skin is largely composed of aerobic
Gram-positive staphylococci and corynebacteria, though anaerobes are
numerous in some areas and Gram-negative bacteria are found in
moister parts. They vary in numbers in different areas between 4000–
400 000 a square centimetre (Noble, 1983). *Staph. aureus* is not often a
resident of healthy dry skin, but it is regularly found in moister parts in
up to 50% of normal individuals, in whom it is often simultaneously
present in the nose.

Resistance to new bacterial colonists (above, p. 12) is a particular
feature of normal skin. This resistance is achieved in co-operation with
the **resident, normal** or **permanent flora**. It is constantly challenged
as parts of the body come into contact with more or less heavily
contaminated surfaces. When foreign bacteria are transferred to the
skin by such contact, some time (perhaps hours) must elapse before
the new temporary residents are disposed of. In the interval, they form

a **transient flora**. One of the most heavily contaminated materials that can act as a donor of transient flora is faeces, followed by the surface of one's own or others' bodies. Ordinary contacts between people, particularly in hospitals, most often involves the hands, so these acquire new transient flora perhaps hundreds of times a day. As long as these very superficial microbes survive, they may be transferred to another individual, again by contact. This is why hands are so important in cross-infection (below, p. 32).

Most of the transient flora is readily removed by ordinary washing. This includes any *Staph. aureus* transferred from individuals own noses to their hands. The importance of this can be determined by watching how often people touch their faces without realizing it. By contrast, the resident flora is much more tenacious, because the microbes concerned spread through the thickness of the cornified layer and down into glands and hair follicles. Washing reduces their number, particularly if disinfectants are used, but the resident flora cannot be removed altogether by any treatment that leaves skin alive. If the skin is damaged or diseased, bacteria that might have been transient may now find conditions suitable for colonization or infection, and so become part of the resident flora. Exposed eczematous skin may harbour a million colonizing *Staph. aureus* per square centimetre, and if the eczema is infected, the number may rise tenfold (Leyden *et al.*, 1974). Hospital staff in this condition are a danger to patients.

Hair has a curiously bad microbiological image. The scale of preoperative shaving that was, and in some places still is, thought necessary is an indication that hair is considered to be an infection hazard. In fact, hair is less able to support microbial multiplication than is the skin from which it grows. Of course, dense hair keeps the underlying skin moist, so encouraging microbial growth. In these circumstances, damp, heavily colonized skin squames separate and are trapped among the hair over it. To this extent, hair is 'dirty', but this does not apply to areas with sparse or short hair, or to hair that is clean. Part of the bad image may be due to the fact that hair and skin squames are both shed, but the result with hair is more obvious and so objectionable. The finding of a hair in the soup is a classical culinary disaster. Fortunately, we are not so easily reminded that every bowl of soup must contain large numbers of invisible squames derived from the skin of the cook who prepared it.

The upper respiratory tract, particularly the mouth and throat, provide a damper, warmer environment in which streptococci are at home. There they are joined by increasing numbers of anaerobic and Gram-negative bacteria. It is popularly supposed that these bacteria escape into the air in large numbers during breathing and speaking and, of course, it is well known that 'coughs and sneezes spread diseases'. In fact, several experiments have shown that many respiratory infections are spread more effectively by such physical contacts as holding a baby or shaking hands (Wenzel *et al.*, 1977; Hall *et al.*, 1980; Couch, 1984). They are spread less effectively by handling items recently used by an infected person, and rather poorly by sitting with them in the same room, with no physical contact. Coughs and sneezes may spread diseases, but the efficiency by which they do so remains in doubt (Anon, 1988) and clouded by arguments that sometimes develop quasi-religious fervour.

The gastrointestinal canal, particularly its lower part, is where much of the normal flora of the body is found. This wet environment lacking oxygen favours anaerobes and many of the Gram-negative rods. Common among the latter is *E. coli*. This bacterium is an even more important cause of HAI than *Staph. aureus*.

The normal flora of the body may change following admission to hospital. How and why this is responsible for self infection with hospital strains of bacteria is described above (p. 12). The growing importance of self-infection in HAI due to various microbes capable of latency is also mentioned above (p. 21). Many of these are viruses, though fungi and protozoa also play a part.

Cross-infection

The microbes responsible for cases of cross-infection are derived directly from the bodies of other people, either patients or staff, or visitors. Because body surfaces are involved these have much in common with, and indeed may be indistinguishable from, cases of self-infection. If they differ at all, they are more likely to be due to hospital strains of bacteria. They may be indistinguishable because it is usually impossible to say if a particular infecting organism was transferred when an infection was initiated or earlier, and so had become part of the patient's normal flora before the infection started. In fact, because a colonization, however brief, must always precede an infection, the distinction between autogenous self-infection and cross-infection is arbitrary. For the reasons noted above, it is believed that hands are the principal vectors in these cases.

Environmental infections

The parts of the environment that may be directly associated with HAI are shown in Figure 2.5. In this diagram, an attempt has been made to distinguish between environmental sources contaminated by man, by

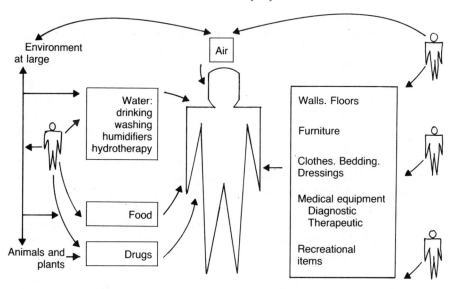

Figure 2.5 A summary of the more important potential sources of environmental infection.

animals or by plants, and the microbes that are derived wholly from the environment.

On its own, the inanimate environment rarely produces microbes that are pathogenic for man. In most cases, it requires the assistance of some other living thing, most often man or sometimes animals or plants. An example of an environmental infection in which the causative microbe may not have been derived from a living thing is legionellosis (legionnaires' disease). Legionellosis is not passed from person to person, and so a patient suffering from it does not need to be isolated to protect other patients or staff. Legionellas grow in water and proliferate actively in certain man-made ecological niches, principally air-conditioning cooling towers and complex plumbing systems. Large modern buildings are particularly vulnerable, and so hospitals have been implicated quite often in outbreaks of the disease. The ecological niche must provide the right temperature (neither too hot nor too cold), plenty of organic matter and a vehicle or vector of infection. In the case of cooling towers, the vector is the fine aerosol of water they spray into the air. If this contains legionellas, they may be inhaled. Although cooling towers are sited on the outside of buildings, the spray from them may be drawn inside through an air intake or a window. Patients in hospital may be exposed to water from contaminated plumbing systems when showering or bathing, or even from water in humidifiers or other respiratory apparatus.

A form of HAI that is more incontrovertibly environmental is aspergillosis. *Aspergillus* spores are ubiquitous, and they have recently emerged as a cause of HAI among the growing population of severely immunocompromised patients. Formerly they were recognized as little more than causes of allergy. Free-living organisms of the *Pseudomonas* and *Acinetobacter* groups grow in damp environmental sites, and may spread from these to cause colonization and perhaps HAI. There is evidence that strains of these bacteria freshly isolated from the environment are less pathogenic than those that have recently caused infections, and so are already adapted to the human body.

Animals (including birds and fishes) and plants are connected to patients as providers of food and less commonly through certain drugs, including the ingredients of some intravenous infusions. Microbes able to cause HAI may pass along the same chain. Many of the standard microbial causes of food poisoning are of animal origin. They are introduced into hospitals in food and regularly cause HAI, in many cases with the active connivance of inefficient kitchens. Animals may also contaminate water supplies. In some tropical countries, insects may be a real problem as vectors of infections like malaria. Such scavengers as semi-wild cats, flies, cockroaches, ants and other winged and creeping arthropods are everywhere perceived to be an infection problem. This reputation is largely undeserved, and it is an interesting example of the confusion that exists in many minds between aesthetic considerations and real causes of infection. In a kitchen, the presence of these pests is an indication of a low standard of hygiene or poor facilities, or both. It is these inadequacies that are the primary causes of food poisoning, and not the pests. They are doing their best to clean up the mess made by dirty humans.

Humans are the most prolific sources of the microbes that cause HAI. Because they are often shed into the environment, it is common to find them in the immediate surroundings of an infected patient, on such things as bedding, floors, furniture and clothing. The question then is to what extent are these microbes capable first of reaching, and second of causing, an infection in another patient?

One of four things may happen to a microbe that has been shed into the environment. Most pathogenic bacteria are accustomed to the five-star accommodation provided for them in or on the human body. In a cold, hard world, they must find alternative sources of nutrition, most critically of water, otherwise most of them die more or less quickly. This is particularly true of the Gram-negative organisms that live on the most sheltered body surface, the gut. Bacteria from drier surfaces of the body withstand desiccation a little better, and so survive longer when they are shed from it. The length of time these organisms take to die varies according to the temperature, humidity, the presence or absence of sunlight, and whether or not they are coated with protective organic matter. For most ordinary bacteria, it is measured in minutes to hours.

The survival of a microbe is not the same as an ability to cause infection. Streptococci that have been exposed to the air for some time can still be grown in the laboratory, but have lost their ability to infect. A number of experiments have been done to prove this, in one of which up to a million living, but partially dried, streptococci were blown directly into the throats of volunteers (Rammelkamp *et al.*, 1964). There were no infections although the same preparations were infectious before they were dried.

Fully virulent streptococci can withstand the attack of poly-morphonuclear leucocytes (PML). These phagocytes are an important part of the body's innate immune system (above, p. 11). Each *Strep. pyogenes* has on its surface one of 70 different kinds of delicate, frond-like proteins, collectively called the 'M' proteins. These act to make the streptococcus resistant to phagocytosis by PML. During an infection, an individual develops antibodies to the M protein of the attacking streptococcus. The next time the individual meets the same strep-tococcus, this antibody neutralizes the M protein and PML can now destroy the attacker. Drying damages the delicate fronds of the M protein, so destroying the organisms' defences against PML. It seems that a desiccated organism is crippled and can no longer infect a surface or tissue where PML are active.

Other bacteria have particular properties that enable them to withstand adverse conditions for a long time. The best examples are the microbes that form seed-like spores. These survive and retain their pathogenicity for months or years without water or nutrients, and can often withstand physical and chemical disinfecting agents as well. This is generally true of the fungi and among bacteria the causes of anthrax, tetanus, botulism, gas gangrene and pseudomembranous colitis are all spore-bearing clostridia. Other bacteria that do not form spores but have similar properties are *Coxiella burnetii* and the tubercle bacillus. The tubercle bacillus may be an important cause of HAI. *C. burnetii* is not.

The pulmonary form of tuberculosis is the common type of this infection. It is caught by inhaling tubercle bacilli (*Mycobacterium tuberculosis*) deep into the lungs. They must reach far down into tor-tuous respiratory passages that are lined by sticky mucus. To achieve this, particles containing the bacilli must be very small, equivalent to about 5 microns in diameter, or less. When coughed up by a person with open tuberculosis, the bacilli are enmeshed in large gobbets of more or less viscous mucus. It is virtually impossible for particles of the size that might cause infections to be formed at this stage. Large wet particles of sputum fall on to the floor or on to other surfaces where they dry and may break up into smaller fragments. If these are swept up into the air, they are available for inhalation and may be of the right size to cause infection. Most microbes trapped in particles of sputum desiccate with the mucus, and so are inactivated or die before they are able to do any harm. Tubercle bacilli are different. They are very resistant to drying, and so survive the process. In this way, viable pathogens are delivered to exactly the right place to establish another tuberculous infection. Tuberculosis is a true environmental infection. Airborne transmission is the principal mode of spread, with man as the source of contamination of the environment. There are not many other examples.

Because it is a common perception that the environment is an important cause of infection, and particularly of HAI, it is necessary to elaborate this point. Reference has been made (Chapter 1) to Semmelweis' evidence that cross-infection is more important than environmental infection as a cause of HAI. Much more recently, the transfer of a teaching hospital to a new building provided confirmation of this. The infection rate among patients and the bacteriological conditions of the two environments were monitored continuously before and after the move. The initially clean environment in the new hospital deteriorated bacteriologically after occupation, taking 6–12 months to reach a state equivalent to the old one. Despite the cleaner environment enjoyed by patients in the first months of occupation of the new hospital, infection rates remained exactly the same (Maki *et al.*, 1982). Another experiment tending to the same conclusion will be described later in the section dealing with wound infections (Chapter 4, p. 68). The principal evidence leading to a contrary view arose from work done in burns units, where conditions are uniquely different (Chapters 4, p. 65 and 6, p. 140).

Perception and reality are at variance in this case, because to establish an infection, a finite and often quite large population of fully virulent microbes must find their way to a portal of entry on a patient. They must then establish a colonization before an infection can develop. Microbes in the environment find this difficult for the reasons just described, but the main reason is numerical. In dry environments (and most of the hospital environment is dry), microbes cannot multiply, and most of them die off more or less quickly. There is an enormous disparity in numbers of bacteria between the dry environment and body surfaces. If the bacteria carried by an average person (10^{15}) were laid one in each of the millimetres that separate the earth and the sun, the line of bacteria would make the round trip all the way there and back about three times. By contrast, the number of bacteria contained in the whole volume of air in a very unsatisfactory operating room (OR) while in use, similarly laid out, would reach the top of a very small hill (about 60 m). The number of bacteria on the floor of the same OR might stretch 5 km, and a floor of similar size that would have been judged hygienically in poor condition when environmental testing was in vogue, might provide enough to stretch 40 km. Confronted by such numerical differences, the logic is inescapable. Self- and cross-infection are far more important causes of HAI than anything that might originate in the dry environment. It is not surprising that applying disinfectants to floors or walls or spraying them into the air has never been proved to be of use.

The situation is totally different for those parts of the environment that are wet. Food and drink are potentially important sources of the bacteria and viruses that may cause HAI. The same applies to drugs used in liquid form. Intravenous infusions, eye drops and disinfecting solutions at 'in use' concentrations all have bad reputations, as do pieces of diagnostic and therapeutic equipment that contain liquid, or that may collect it in the form of condensation. These are all potential sources of infection as there are obvious vectors or vehicles that connect them to patients. These and other examples of environmental hazards associated with wet environments are considered again in Chapter 6 (p. 141). Precautions quite properly applied to prevent harm in these cases should not be extended without thought to other areas. Once more it is necessary to make a distinction between sources and reservoirs. For instance, disinfectants poured down drains are wasted, and needlessly contaminate the environment.

SURVEYS AND TRIALS

A survey is used to find out how many infections there are in a hospital and to locate them. Surveys are an expensive waste of time if the results are not put to good use. When one is contemplated, the first action is to define why it is needed. A short list of reasons for studying infections in hospital might include a wish to raise awareness of the existence of such infections among those who have ignored them, as a first step in the process of control; to identify areas where infections are more common as a preliminary to more detailed study; to measure the effect of control measures and justify expenditure on them; and, in some parts of the world, to use the data collected as a defence in litigation. The initial definition is doubly important because the reason for making a survey shapes the decisions that follow. Some surveys are designed to discover facts – the numbers of infections and where they are, for instance. Surveys that set out to make comparisons and determine choices, as when groups of patients are subjected to different treatments, are usually called trials.

The next decision is to choose the type of study to be made. The choice is between an **incidence** and a **prevalence** approach. A prevalence survey involves counting the number of patients with infections in the population at the time of the study. Depending on how many patients are to be included, their geographical distribution and the number of individuals making the survey, it will usually be completed in one or just a few days. As each infection is found, its site and type are recorded together with any other information required. The effect of this is to take a snapshot of the community, frozen at the time of the survey. An incidence survey is similar, but it is conducted over a significant period, or it may be continuous. As the population surveyed changes with time, this approach produces a video film compared with the still photograph of a prevalence study. Because patients with infections stay in hospital longer, at any one time they occupy a disproportionately large number of beds. A prevalence survey will, therefore, record more cases of infection than an incidence study, in which the unit is a single patient, no matter how long he or she stays in hospital. This is why rates of infection determined by prevalence surveys are higher than are found in incidence studies. This does not matter provided the results are not directly compared with each other. Incidence studies are the 'gold standard', but they are time-consuming, labour intensive and expensive. Prevalence surveys are quick and cheaper to perform. Whichever type of survey is chosen, and unless it is small, a pilot study involving a few patients should be held to test the methods to be used. This allows any errors or omissions to be corrected before starting the survey proper.

Next, the population to be surveyed must be defined. This might be anything from the patients in a single ward or other small unit, to all of those in a number of hospitals in a region or country, or even in several countries. In making the decision, one of the key factors will be the size of the problem to be measured. It is no use surveying ten patients to discover something about an infection that happens only once in every 100 of them. This is obvious, and for a simple survey of infection in hospitals common sense will be a good guide to the size of the population needed. The problem is different when comparisons are to be made, and the rate of a certain event is to be measured and

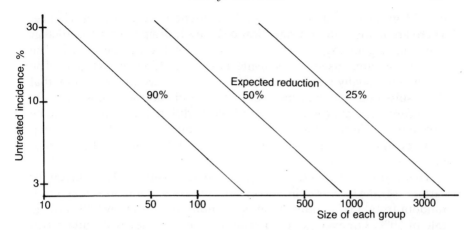

Figure 2.6 The sizes of test and control groups needed to establish a statistically significant result under varying conditions of incidence of the condition under study in the control group, and the reduction in this incidence expected as a result of intervention in the test group (for an even chance at the 5% level). (Drawn from data by Lidwell, O. M. (1963)).

compared in test and control groups. If the event is common, and the procedure to be tested very effective, the groups can be quite small. When Lister introduced antiseptic surgery, a rate of mortality of 46% in his control group of amputees was reduced to 15% in the antiseptic test group. Control and test groups of 35 and 40 were sufficient to prove the point statistically; that is, for the figures to stand up to mathematical analysis using an appropriate statistical test. Figure 2.6 shows how the size of the groups needed to produce significant results grow as the incidence of the event to be measured falls and the expected difference between test and control groups diminishes. When planning an important study, expert statistical help is essential to avoid the chance of making an expensive mistake.

The last decision before detailed planning begins is the choice of the criteria or definitions to be used. In the case of infections in hospitals, it will be necessary to define precisely each of the types of infection to be counted, and so there will be no argument later about what exactly was meant, for instance, by a wound infection. It is usual to adopt a set of definitions that have already been used by someone else, both to avoid making mistakes, and to allow the results to be compared with those of others. A part of this process will be to decide who will perform the survey, what information to collect and how to gather it.

At the end of a trial it is usually necessary to apply a statistical test to the results, to determine if any difference observed between test and control groups is 'significant', or if it might have arisen by chance. There are many different statistical tests, each designed for a particular situation. Again expert help is necessary for the inexperienced. The tests most often used in medicine have one thing in common. The calculation usually results in a figure that estimates the probability that the results of any two or more of the test and control samples that are to be compared are (or are not) sufficiently different for the result to be declared significant. Put another way, the question is asked if the gap between the results is (or is not) so great that it could not (or could) have been due to chance.

This can be illustrated by imagining that a search is to be made for carriers of *Staph. aureus* in successive groups of four nurses taken at random from a large number among whom there is an overall carriage rate of 50%. On average, each sample of four nurses will contain two with positive and two with negative culture results but, of course, as testing continues any of the following 16 variations are possible (+ denotes a positive and − a negative).

					Chances
No positives	− − − −				1/16
One positive	+ − − −	− + − −	− − + −	− − − +	4/16 (1/4)
Two positives	+ + − −	+ − + −	− − + +		
	− + − +	− + + −	+ − − +		6/16 (3/8)
Three positives	+ + + −	+ − + +	+ + − +	− + + +	4/16 (1/4)
Four positives	+ + + +				1/16

The probability of all four nurses in a group being negative (or positive) is 1/16. The probability of only one of them being negative (or positive) is 4/16 or 1/4, and that of there being equal numbers negative and positive is 6/16 or 3/8. Notice that the fractions add up to 1, which is the probability (certainty) that four nurses were tested at a time. The value for the probability (the 'p' value) of certainty is 1, and that of an impossibility is 0. The nearer the value of p gets to 1, the more likely it is that an event will take place, or that groups being compared are the same. The closer p is to 0, the more likely it is that it will not, or that the groups are significantly different. A p value of 0.5 means that probabilities are 50:50, like those of a coin coming down heads. To calculate p from the fractions above, the upper figure of each fraction is divided by the lower, giving values of 0.06, 0.25 and 0.38. Some prefer to express chances in percentages, when $p = 1 = 100\%$. The fractions then become 6, 25 and 38%, respectively.

The value of p that can be accepted as denoting a significant difference lies next to the one that might be due to chance. The choice of figure is arbitrary. The least demanding convention is to say that if a given observation would happen by chance once in 20 otherwise identical trials, or less often than that (p = 0.05 or a chance of 5%, or less), the difference is significant. A more demanding test of significance is to say that the observation would happen by chance once in 100 trials or less often (p = 0.01 or 1%, or less).

This can be illustrated by referring once more to Lister's results. The 'chi squared' test is a simple but appropriate one to apply in this case. Calculation gives a p value of between 0.005 (0.5%) and 0.001 (0.1%), so a difference in mortality between control (precarbolic) and test (carbolic) groups as large as that observed would be found due to chance once in rather more than 200 trials. The probability that the results of Lister's single experiment were due to luck is equivalent to having a coin come down 'heads' eight or nine times in succession. This is highly unlikely, so the conclusion is that the improvement was due to the disinfectant.

The results of a trial may be used to validate a new infection control policy, or to justify a change in an established one. The replacement of unvalidated rituals by scientifically planned policies is to be applauded, but a word of caution is necessary when changes are to be made as a result of studies performed in other places. Endemic HAI is a mixture of self-, cross- and environmental infections (Chapter 2, p. 28). Call these A, B and C, and assume that for a particular type of infection, B is generally the more common cause. If a trial is done in a hospital in which B is already well controlled, an improvement will be noted if measures to reduce the effect of A or C are tested. If these apparently successful control measures are then transferred to a hospital where infections are still more common because B is poorly controlled, little or no improvement will result. This is because type B infections continue unchecked, and their greater number may swamp any small improvement due to the control of factors A or C. This is one reason why published results of trials of infection control procedures may conflict.

FURTHER READING

Martin, S. M. (1968) Statistical considerations for analysis of nosocomial infection data, in *Hospital Infections*, 2nd edn, (eds J. V. Bennett and P. S. Brachman), Little Brown, Boston, pp. 95–111.

Wardlaw, A. C. (1985) *Practical Statistics for Experimental Biologists*, John Wiley, Chichester.

REFERENCES

Anon (1988) Splints don't stop colds – surprising! *Lancet*, **i**, 277–8.

Bernander, S., Habraeus, A., Myrback, K. E. *et al.* (1978) Prevalence of hospital-acquired infections in five Swedish hospitals in November 1975. *Scand. J. Infect. Dis.*, **10**, 66–70.

Casewell, M. W. and Phillips, I. (1978) Epidemiological patterns of klebsiella colonization and infection in an intensive care ward. *J. Hyg., Camb.*, **80**, 295–300.

Chow, A. W., Taylor, P. R., Yoshikawa, T. T., *et al.* (1979) A nosocomial outbreak of infections due to multiply resistant *Proteus mirabilis*: role of intestinal colonization as a major reservoir. *J. Infect. Dis.*, **139**, 621–27.

Couch, R. B. (1984) The common cold: control? *J. Infect. Dis.*, **150**, 167–73.

Cross, A., Allen, J. R., Burke, J., *et al.* (1983) Nosocomial infections due to *Pseudomonas aeruginosa*: review of recent trends. *Rev. Infect. Dis.*, **5** (Supplement 5), 837–45.

Curie, K., Speller, D. C. E., Simpson, R. A., *et al.* (1978) A hospital epidemic caused by a gentamicin-resistant *Klebsiella aerogenes*. *J. Hyg., Camb.*, **80**, 115–23.

Edman, J. C., Kovacs, J. A., Masur, H., *et al.* (1988) Ribosomal RNA sequence shows *Pneumocystis carinii* to be a member of the fungi. *Nature*, **334**, 519–22.

Elek, S. D. and Conen, P. E. (1957) The virulence of *Staphylococcus pyogenes* for man. A study of the problems of wound infection. *Brit. J. Exp. Path.*, **38**, 573–86.

French, G. L., Cheng, A. and Farrington, M. (1987) Prevalence survey of infection in a Hong Kong hospital using a standard protocol and microcomputer analysis. *J. Hosp. Infect.*, **9**, 132–42.

Goldman, D. A. (1986) Epidemiology of *Staphylococcus aureus* and group A streptococci, in *Hospital Infections*, 2nd edn, (eds J. V. Bennett and P. S. Brachman), Little Brown, Boston, pp. 483–94.

Haley, R. W. (1986) Incidence and nature of endemic and epidemic nosocomial infections, in *Hospital Infections*, 2nd edn, (eds J. V. Bennett and P. S. Brachman), Little Brown, Boston, pp. 359–74.

Hall, C. B., Douglas, R. G. and Geiman, J. M. (1980) Possible transmission by fomites of respiratory syncytial virus. *J. Infect. Dis.*, **141**, 98–102.

Hinton, N. A. (1976) Incidence and character of nosocomial infectious diseases, in *Diagnosis and Management of Gram-Negative Nosocomial Diseases*, (eds I. B. R. Duncan, N. A. Hinton and J. O. Godden), Medi-Edit, Toronto, pp. 1–12.

Hovig, B., Lystad, A. and Opsjon, H. (1981) A prevalence survey of infections among hospitalized patients in Norway. *Natl Inst. Pub. Hlth (Oslo) Annals*, **4**, 49–60.

Jepsen, O. B. and Mortensen, N. (1980) Prevalence of nosocomial infections and infection control in Denmark. *J. Hosp. Inf.*, **1**, 237–44.

Kislak, J. W., Eickhoff, T. C. and Finland, M. (1964) Hospital acquired infections and antibiotic usage in the Boston City Hospital – January 1964. *New Eng. J. Med.*, **271**, 834–5.

Leyden, J. J., Marples, R. R. and Kligman, A. M. (1974) *Staphylococcus aureus* in the lesions of atopic dermatitis. *Brit. J. Dermatol.*, **90**, 525–30.

Lidwell, O. M. (1963) Methods of Investigation and Analysis of Results in *Infection in Hospitals* (eds R. E. O. Williams and R. A. Shooter). Blackwell, Oxford, p. 45.

Maki, D. G., Alvarado, C. J., Hassemer, C. A. *et al.* (1982) Relation of the inanimate environment to endemic nosocomial infection. *New Eng. J. Med.*, **307**, 1562–6.

Meers, P. D., Ayliffe, G. A. J., Emmerson, A. M. *et al.* (1981) Report on the national survey of infection in hospitals, 1980. *J. Hosp. Infect.*, **2** (Supplement), 1–53.

Meers, P. D. and Leong, K. Y. (1990) The impact of methicillin- and aminoglycoside-resistant *Staphylococcus aureus* on the pattern of hospital-acquired infection in an acute hospital. *J. Hosp. Infect.*, **16**, 231–39.

Meers, P. D. and Yeo, G. A. (1978) Shedding of bacteria and skin squames after handwashing. *J. Hyg., Camb.*, **81**, 99–105.

Moro, M. L., Stazi, M. A., Marasca, G. *et al.* (1986) National prevalence survey of hospital-acquired infections in Italy, 1983. *J. Hosp. Infect.*, **8**, 72–85.

Noble, W. C. (1983) Microbiology of normal skin, in *Microbial Skin Disease: its Epidemiology*, (ed. W. C. Noble), Edward Arnold, London, pp. 4–15.

Pitt, T. L., Erdman, Y. J. and Bucher, C. (1980) The epidemiological type identification of *Serratia marcescens* from outbreaks of infection in hospitals. *J. Hyg., Camb.*, **84**, 269–83.

Rammelkamp, C. H., Mortimer, E. A. and Wolinsky, E. (1964) Transmission of streptococcal and staphylococcal infections. *Ann. Int. Med.*, **60**, 753–8.

Scheckler, W., Garner, J. S., Kaiser, A. B. *et al.* (1971) Prevalence of infections and antibiotic usage in eight community hospitals, in *Proceedings of the International Conference on Nosocomial Infections*, (eds P. S. Brachman and T. C. Eickhoff), American Hospital Association, Chicago, pp. 299–305.

Selwyn, S. and Ellis, H. (1972) Skin bacteria and skin disinfection reconsidered. *Brit. Med. J.*, **1**, 136–40.

Shanson, D. C. (1981) Antibiotic-resistant *Staphylococcus aureus*. *J. Hosp. Infect.*, **2**, 11–36.

Wenzel, R. P., Deal, E. C. and Hendley, J. O. (1977) Hospital-acquired viral respiratory illness on a pediatric ward. *Pediatrics*, **60**, 367–71.

Part Two

Control of infection in hospitals

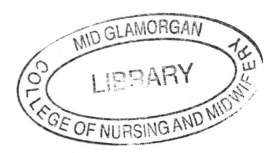

Chapter 3

Introduction to, history, and the organization and delivery of infection control

INTRODUCTION AND HISTORY

For patients that enter them, hospitals are dangerous places. A number will die, and some will suffer from an accident while they are there. Accidents may be physical (falling out of bed or an overdose of radiation, for example), medical (wrong drug, wrong dose, wrong operation or a technical error), psychological (reaction to stress) or patients may acquire an infection. Florence Nightingale said that at the very least, hospitals should do the sick no harm. Although this absolute is unachievable, health professionals have a duty to approach it as closely as possible. The safe delivery of health care is an important objective.

The best estimates of the human and financial impact of infections acquired in hospitals (HAI, Chapter 2, p. 16) come from the USA. It has been estimated that between 5 and 6% of patients who were admitted to US hospitals in the 1970s and early 1980s suffered at least one HAI, amounting to some two million cases a year. Each year about 20 000 people died as a direct result of HAI, and HAI contributed to a further 60 000 deaths. On average an infected patient spent an extra four days in hospital. The additional cost in 1985 was just over $1800 each for an annual total of $3.9 billion, excluding the cost of associated litigation (Haley, 1986). Pain and anxiety cannot be quantified.

An unknown proportion of HAI is avoidable (Chapter 2, p. 14). The US Study on the Efficacy of Nosocomial Infection Control (SENIC) showed that a properly conducted programme of surveillance and control can prevent 32% or nearly one-third of cases. It has been estimated that the control programme necessary to produce this result would be self-financing if 6% of infections were prevented (Haley and Garner, 1986). A reduction of 32% represents a handsome profit on the investment. The return in human terms is incalculable. Infection control can be very cost effective. Cost efficiency may be improved even further if wasteful rituals are excluded.

It is difficult to date the beginnings of attempts to control infections in hospitals. Hospitals specializing in major community acquired infections, such as smallpox and yellow fever, were already in existence at the beginning of the eighteenth century. By this time, venereal diseases were being treated in isolation annexes of hospitals called 'Locks'. At the beginning of the twentieth century, fever hospitals abounded, and rules for their management represent early attempts to control infection in hospitals. Fever hospitals began to close in the mid-twentieth century as the number of patients requiring admission fell; in most places those specializing in tuberculosis were the last to disappear. As a result, cases of classical infections that needed to be admitted had to go to ordinary acute hospitals. To prevent the spread of infection to other patients, methods formerly employed in fever hospitals were introduced into general hospitals. These included barrier nursing.

An early suggestion for an ordered approach to the control of hospital as distinct from community acquired infection was contained in a 1941 memorandum from the UK Medical Research Council. In response to concern about infection in wartime surgical wounds this recommended that hospitals appoint 'full time officers to supervise the control of infection'. In 1944, the same organization proposed that every hospital should set up a committee representing doctors, nurses, laboratory workers and administrators to investigate and design measures to control all forms of HAI. These separate ideas were brought together at the time of the 80/81 staphylococcal pandemic (Chapter 2, p. 25), and in 1959 hospitals were advised to set up infection control committees (ICCs) as well as to appoint control of infection officers (CIOs). In 1959 in Torbay, England Miss E. M. Cottrell was appointed as the first infection control nurse (ICN) (Meers, 1980). Infection control had by then begun to appear as a regular topic for discussion at scientific meetings, and as the subject of publications.

These developments were mirrored in the USA, where the initial stimulus was also the 80/81 staphylococcus. A training course for ICNs was set up in 1968, and the first of a series of International Conferences on Nosocomial Infections was held in 1970. The Centers for Disease Control (CDC) provided strong central leadership backed up by research, and further interest was generated by the publication of an infection control manual by the American Hospital Association. The surveillance and control of HAI became an important preoccupation in many American hospitals.

During the 1970s and 1980s, there was a proliferation of books, manuals, journals and professional associations concerned with the control of HAI. The Infection Control Nurses' Association (ICNA) set up in the UK in 1970 was joined in 1972 by the Association for

Practitioners of Infection Control (APIC) in the USA. The UK-based Hospital Infection Society was established in 1979, and the Society of Hospital Epidemiologists of America was formed in 1980. By this time HAI and its control had acquired all the features of a new medical sub-speciality.

ORGANIZATION

The skills required by those attempting to control HAI are a knowledge of the diagnosis, microbiology, epidemiology, treatment and control of infectious disease, in the hospital setting. A sound knowledge of the geography and administrative structure of their own hospital is a necessity, as is an ability to communicate effectively with staff at all levels, individually or in groups. The availability of time to do the job and the patience to see it through are final prerequisites. Many of these skills and talents may be found in medically qualified microbiologists and infectious disease physicians, providing they have had training in HAI. When available, such people ought to be appointed as CIOs. Because they have other duties, one or more ICNs are usually employed to support them. The combination produces a small but highly effective infection control team (ICT).

An ICT normally reports to, and is monitored by, an ICC. An ICC should have among its members senior administrative personnel from all the main departments of the hospital, plus influential clinicians from the major specialities. The chairperson should be a senior member of the hospital staff, who has, or who commands, executive authority. Unless a CIO possesses this authority, he or she should not be chairperson. Indeed, it can be argued that such an appointment leads to a CIO monitoring him or herself. The ICC needs to meet regularly to support a newly formed ICT, or when for some reason an established team is in difficulty. An experienced and effective team requires to be monitored less often, and the ICC may then only meet to deal with large problems or make major policy decisions.

To be effective an ICT must co-ordinate three functions. These are summarized in Figure 3.1 as input, digestion and output activities. Input is of two kinds, routine and occasional. Routine input is the regular accumulation of information on infections present in a hospital. This is an active process if it involves one or more members of the team in a direct search for cases of infection, or it is passive if notifications result from the actions of others. These approaches are described below. Occasional input consists of questions on matters concerned with the control of infection directed to members of the team. Some

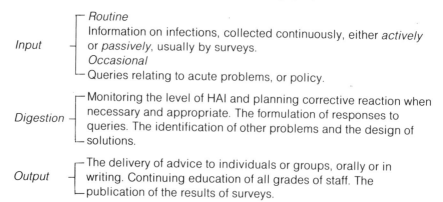

Figure 3.1 A flow-chart summarizing the functions of an infection control team in a hospital.

queries require immediate responses, for example, what to do about a patient with an unexpected infection problem, or the action to take when a vital machine breaks down. Other questions are more general, as might arise from the introduction of a new fibreoptic diagnostic or therapeutic tool that requires modification of an existing sterilization and disinfection policy. Another example would be an infection control contribution to plans for the establishment of a new oncology or transplant unit. Enquiries of these kinds may come from medical or nursing staff, or from members of the support services. Of the latter administration, central sterile supply, pharmacy, catering, domestic and laundry services provide the largest number of queries, but every department in the hospital eventually makes contact with the ICT. A courteous and helpful response to queries, even if repetitive and seemingly pointless, is the hallmark of an effective team.

In the USA, a systematic national system was developed based on active surveillance for the collection of routine input data. In its complete form, this requires ICNs (nurse-epidemiologists) to spend a significant amount of time in a search for infections. Every day the results of cultures sent to microbiology laboratories are scrutinized, X-ray departments and wards are visited to locate patients whose films suggest infection, or whose charts indicate a fever, the use of antimicrobials or the application of isolation precautions. Records are kept and periodic summaries are produced and circulated. A continuous incidence survey of this sort (Chapter 2, p. 38) occupies one full-time nurse with clerical support for every 250 beds served. This expensive approach is justified if something useful is done with the data collected.

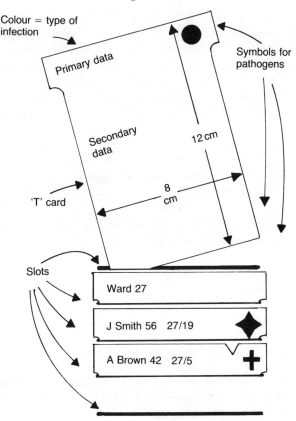

Figure 3.2 Illustration of 'T' cards to show their approximate size and shape. These can be cut out of stiff card if the commercially made ones are not available. The colour of the card (four or more different colours may be used) indicates the type of infection, say, yellow for UTI, red for SWI, etc. Alternatively, a single colour may be used with coloured adhesive flashes to indicate the infection. Stick-on motifs of different colours and shapes indicate the six or seven most common pathogens. A variety of these motifs can be found in stationery stores. The primary data describes the patient and his or her location, the secondary will include such things as date of admission and eventually of discharge, clinical diagnosis, antibiogram of the pathogen, date of surgery, catheterization and so on, according to the wishes of the ICT. It is a good idea to include cases of significant CAI on the board, particularly if transmission of the infection within the hospital is possible. This makes the origin of such spread obvious. To avoid confusing CAI with HAI, a notch may be cut in the top of the card (see the lowest card in the illustration). The slotted board used to hold the cards, made of pressed steel sections, is available from suppliers of office equipment. Sufficient of these sections are joined together so that each ward or other clinical area is allocated an area of its own, comprising 8–10 slots.

In other places, the search for cases of HAI is initiated by persons who do not belong to the team, so for the ICT the collection of data is a passive process. Information is derived mainly from one source, usually and most effectively from the microbiology laboratory. Any culture result that suggests an infection is followed up by the ICN, who visits the ward to distinguish between colonization and infection (Chapter 2, p. 14) and for infections between those acquired in the community and the hospital. In the case of HAI, other relevant details are collected. At the same time, the opportunity is taken to talk to the staff to discover problems and disseminate information. When visits are complete, the ICN returns to base (ideally in or near the laboratory) to log the information collected. A powerful way of making and displaying these records is to use the 'T' cards and a slotted board illustrated in Figure 3.2. This system makes the detection of clusters of similar infections or of infections due to the same microbe a matter of simple observation. The system allows information to be updated daily in a way that relates microbial pathogens, sites of infection and the clinical areas involved in a visually easily assimilated fashion, instantly accessible to anyone who needs to know about it. At the end of the month, cards that refer to patients who have been discharged are removed from the board. The information they carry is stored in whatever format is preferred; at the simplest level they are filed in a box.

Computers can replace T cards and boards. The strength of a computer is that periodic statements can be extracted and special surveys made with minimum additional effort. Its weakness is that the recognition of an outbreak (and any corrective action that might be necessary) is delayed unless data entry and full file interrogation are performed daily. Computer print-outs require knowledgeable interpretation, and so information may not be available to all who need it. Some people find a stack of ten or 20 computer print-outs incomprehensible.

Periodic extraction of information from T cards into a more compact format (including but not necessarily by computer) yields data that can be converted into a continuous incidence study of HAI. When information is derived from one source only, the survey is incomplete. If laboratory requests are used as the principal source, the proportion of all HAI detected depends on the frequency of microbiological sampling among infections diagnosed clinically. This proportion is usually unknown, and so the total incidence of HAI cannot be estimated. Rarely sampling may approach 100%, but it is nearly always lower. In NUH (Chapter 2, p. 18) it was estimated at between one-third and a half. Despite this deficiency, information that is carefully and consistently collected gives data that are comparable over months and years with regard to the proportion of all HAI sampled, its types and distribution, and its microbial causes. A change in one or more of these measures calls for investigation. An experienced ICN properly integrated into a microbiology laboratory can perform this kind of incomplete incidence study for about 600 beds and, perhaps, more, with time to spare for other infection control duties. Other forms of incomplete incidence study can be imagined. For example, intensive care units might be subjected to a continuous complete survey, with sporadic activity directed at other areas in rotation, perhaps using prevalence studies as described below. Of course, a continuous watch is maintained for evidence of unusual infection anywhere in the hospital. This duty falls primarily to the person who signs or otherwise validates laboratory reports before they are released.

In hospitals with rudimentary microbiology services, or where such a service is lacking, other sources of routine input data must be found if anything is to be done at all. This can take the form of regular, usually weekly, returns made by the staff of each ward or clinical department. On this are listed cases of HAI that have been noted. The standard form designed for this purpose should not require so much detail that this alone will deter those who should complete it. Information derived in this way is usually of poor quality, but it provides a crude measure of events when records from each area are compared week by week, and in any case it is nearly always better than nothing.

There is another approach to the acquisition of routine input data. Laboratory based studies as just described may be used for day-to-day surveillance of infections. These are then supplemented by periodic prevalence surveys (Chapter 2, p. 38), involving either a whole hospital or selected departments. Prevalence surveys are quick and cheap to perform. They can detect changes in the prevalence of one or other kind of HAI, and so can be used to monitor the effect of new policies, or to discover how and why antimicrobial drugs are being prescribed. They are a good way of impressing hospital staff with the importance of HAI.

As described in Chapter 2, p. 39, before any kind of survey can begin the various types of infection to be counted must be defined. Examples of definitions are given in the Appendix (p. 167). Definitions ought to be simple and memorable. Over-sophistication is self-defeating, particularly where infection control activity is poorly developed, and when returns of infections are completed by ward staff.

Members of an experienced ICT are able to respond to many of the questions they are asked immediately, because they have met and

Table 3.1 An outline of the elements that make up a service for the control of infection in hospitals

---

Set up an infection control team
(plus an infection control committee to monitor it)

to conduct a **surveillance programme**, provide **advice**
and **react** to **problems**, and to contribute to the formulation of

policies (antimicrobial, disinfection and sterilization, isolation
laundry, waste, staff vaccination and safety, etc.)

and

procedures when using catheters (urinary and IV) or ventilators,
or performing dressings, etc.

and

to monitor the provision of

adequate facilities for handwashing, sterile supply, and in
operating departments, isolation rooms, kitchens, etc.

---

dealt with the same problem before. New problems require 'digestion' (Table 3.1), during which a solution is agreed in discussion between members of the ICT. Without consensus, the output of a team is likely to be inconsistent. Any advice then lacks credibility, and so is ignored. The method employed to reach decisions vary with the knowledge and experience of team members, but this book and others like it are designed to assist the process.

At one time, many ICTs involved themselves in a significant amount of bacteriological monitoring of the environment. Floors, walls, the air, water, food, medications and disinfectants might all be sampled on a routine basis, and sterilizers checked for their ability to kill bacterial spores. Most of these activities have been abandoned as unhelpful, other than when clearly indicated as a part of the investigation of an outbreak of infection. Routine checks may still be carried out (perhaps weekly) on infant feeds prepared in hospital milk kitchens, or on hospital water supplies if these are of doubtful quality. The testing of sterilizers is discussed in Chapter 5 (p. 111).

DELIVERY

Information emerges from ICTs as **advice**. CIOs and ICNs should rarely if ever be given executive authority. In clinical matters, final authority belongs to those with full responsibility for patients, and this cannot be usurped or easily shared without threatening their welfare. More practically, there can be no output from an ICT that lacks input. Potential contributors of input may withhold it if they cannot exert some control over the action that might follow. It is important to remember that advice concerning infection control is only one of a number of often competing and, perhaps, mutually exclusive factors that must be considered in reaching decisions in hospitals.

The output from an effective ICT ranges over nearly all hospital activity. It is likely to include contributions to long-term building and operational plans, the use of disinfectants and antimicrobials, the management of areas with particular infection problems, such as dialysis, transplant, oncology and intensive care units. Other topics on which advice is given include the disposal of waste, methods used for cleaning, or the handling of laundry apart from more obvious areas, such as patient isolation, the testing of autoclaves and the safety of food.

Much advice may be consolidated into written procedures and policies (Table 3.1). It would be possible to divide all hospital activity into a large number of brief individual procedures, each recorded in a step-by-step fashion. The result would be confusing, repetitious, difficult to co-ordinate and probably ignored, and so wasteful. However, certain discrete activities, particularly in the nursing field, are best handled in this way. This allows infection control advice to be included in procedures for dressing wounds or caring for catheters, tracheostomies or central venous lines, for instance. In other cases, advice is best incorporated into policies. These describe the basis for certain activities that are related by common factors, such as the choice and use of an economical set of multipurpose disinfectants, the need, and methods, for patient isolation, dealing with laundry or the handling of waste. A disinfectant policy, for instance, may include everything from the preparation of the skin for a variety of different procedures, to the methods to be used for cleaning and disinfecting endoscopes.

Each hospital should decide which activities they wish to co-ordinate, and how these should be divided between procedures and policies. The necessary administrative structures are then devised to ensure that everyone who should be, is consulted. This is important to secure compliance. For instance, when writing procedures a nursing procedures committee ought to seek advice from the ICN (or from the ICT or ICC through the ICN) on matters relating to the control of infection. For activities that involve wider sections of the hospital community, the ICC or some other appropriate body may set up subcommittees or small *ad hoc* bodies to devise the necessary policies. These should have powers of co-option so that, for instance, an endoscopist is involved when the cleaning and disinfection of endoscopes is discussed.

Information is disseminated in a variety of ways. An effective ICT has to develop lines of communication to a larger number of individuals and groups in a hospital than anyone else, administration excepted. An effective team must be able to identify, reach and influence those who make executive decisions, from the least to the most important. This involves many visits, much talking, and a lot of shoe leather.

Most acute questions are answered face to face, or by telephone. Less acute matters and policies are handled differently, and the method will vary with the administrative structure of the hospital. When administrative power is vested in a single individual or a small group, advice is best channelled through an ICC, particularly if the chairperson is a powerful figure. In hospitals in which power is more diffuse, committees proliferate, and user bodies may have considerable influence. Most of these groups will at some time hold discussions that impinge on infection and its control. An ICT should be prepared for its members to be co-opted to such committees on these occasions, to help make cost-effective decisions and, perhaps, prevent costly mistakes.

An important part of advice giving is education. This may be used in two ways. The publication of infection surveillance data ought to educate those who receive it. Unfortunately, it all too often ends up unread in the waste-paper basket. One method that has been used to attract attention is to publish it so that recipients recognize their own contribution to HAI without this being obvious to anyone else. This approach has reduced the incidence of surgical wound infections (Chapter 4, p. 69). The second application of education is to orient staff to an awareness of the existence of an infection problem, and their role in the control of it. This should be done formally during the education of doctors and nurses, with periodic in-service refresher courses. Other employees should be taught the principles of infection control as applied to their own work on first appointment, again with refreshers from time to time. The elements of a complete infection control programme are summarized in Table 3.1.

Throughout their careers, many doctors will spend more time dealing with infections than with any other organic disease. It is surprising that medical schools in general spend so little time educating medical undergraduates in a subject that will occupy so much of their working lives. So far as HAI is concerned, this may not even be mentioned in an undergraduate course. Although nurses will be taught about the prevention of infection, tutors in schools of nursing are unlikely to have received any formal education in the developing science of hospital infection control. Some recognize this and use a qualified ICN to make up the deficiency, unfortunately others do not. The result is that wasteful and illogical ritual is taught, much of it based on ideas current 20 to 30 years ago, that were sometimes wrong even then.

The requirement for a formal programme to monitor and control HAI is directly attributable to this dual failure of education. Health care is delivered to individual patients by individual doctors and nurses. The safety of its delivery and, in particular, the avoidance of infection is determined at the same level. The requirement that doctors and nurses should be monitored in this part of their overall work is a measure of how serious the failure is. The problem should be tackled at its foundation. The object should be to make ICNs redundant or, more positively, make all nurses their own ICNs. In the developed parts of the world, inertia in the existing system makes this a distant prospect. Paradoxically, it might be more easily achieved in less-developed areas. Where infection control programmes are themselves only ideas, a relatively minor expenditure on education would have a disproportionately large effect.

The average physician or surgeon tends to a heavy commitment to the patient of the moment, and gives little thought to them in groups. Nurses, although also oriented to individual patients, **are** trained to care for them in groups. Although infection control rests on an intimate triangular relationship between each patient, nurse and doctor, Table 3.1 shows that infection control behaviour is determined by group decisions. Not only are nurses more likely to react positively to these, but they are more numerous and they come into intimate contact with patients more often than other hospital staff. Of course, both doctors and nurses should be better educated, but this analysis suggests that effort directed at nurses will produce the greater return more quickly. The points at which maximum benefit can result from minimum input is in medical schools and schools of nursing, with the emphasis on the latter. Education of the educators is the key and, as with all wisdom, the recognition of ignorance is the first step.

REFERENCES

Haley, R. W. (1986) Incidence and nature of endemic and epidemic nosocomial infections, in *Hospital Infections*, 2nd edn (eds J. V. Bennett and P. S. Brachman) Little Brown, Boston, pp. 359–74.

Haley, R. W. and Garner, J. S. (1986) Infection surveillance and control programs, in *Hospital Infections*, 2nd edn (eds J. V. Bennett and P. S. Brachman) Little Brown, Boston, pp. 39–50.

Meers, P. D. (1980) The organisation of infection control in hospitals. *J. Hosp. Infect.*, **1**, 187–91.

Chapter 4

The different infections

URINARY TRACT INFECTIONS

With some uniformity, surveys have shown that urinary tract infections (UTI) are the most common form of HAI (Chapter 2, p. 18), accounting for between 30% and 45% of it. To highlight the features that determine this dominance and as an aid to comprehension, some numerical data are given below. These have been taken from a variety of sources, and so the picture that emerges is a composite one (unless otherwise noted see reviews by Stamm, 1986; Stickler, 1990; Warren, 1990).

The association between infections of the urinary tract and urethral catheterization (thought to be the cause of about 80% of hospital acquired UTI) and other forms of urethral instrumentation (about 10%) is very strong. In a prevalence study, 21% of patients who were catheterized had UTI compared with only 3% of those who were not. The same study found overall that, at any one time 10% of patients in acute general hospitals were catheterized, with a higher proportion among the elderly (Meers *et al.*, 1981). The duration of catheterization varies, but another study showed that half had been removed by the fourth day, and 80% were out by the tenth day (Mulhall *et al.*, 1988). With closed drainage (Figure 4.1) and average conditions of care, just under 10% of uninfected patients are newly infected each day catheterization persists, reaching a total of 50–60% by the tenth day. Rates of acquisition above this should be investigated because it is likely that serious mistakes are being made. Lower rates do not call for congratulation until figures of 20–30% at ten days are achieved. On open drainage, almost 100% of catheterized patients are colonized or infected by the fourth day. With well-managed closed systems, the 100% level is not reached until about the 30th day.

Septicaemia is the most serious complication of UTI, reported in between 1% and 3% of cases. Septicaemia has a mortality of 30% or

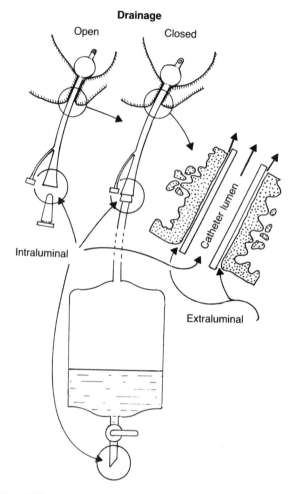

Figure 4.1 The difference between open and closed drainage of the urinary tract, and the points at which microbes gain access to it.

more. The high frequency of catheter-related UTI pushes the urinary catheter firmly into the spotlight as a major cause of death due to HAI.

With the exception of the distal part of the urethra, the healthy urinary tract is sterile. The distal part of the urethra is colonized by members of the normal flora of the perineum, which includes bacteria from the gut. Periodic voiding and the constant flow of urine into the bladder restricts the upward spread of colonization, and this is aided by the secretion of bactericidal substances from the prostate in the male and the periurethral glands in the female.

Bacteria can grow in urine. Lister used urine as his culture medium when he repeated Pasteur's experiment that disproved the spontaneous generation of life (Chapter 1, p. 5). Urine is inanimate and so cannot itself be infected, but a sufficiently heavy colonization leads in time to inflammatory changes in the lining of the urinary tract, and so to UTI. The urinary tract is most commonly invaded from below through the urethra (ascending infection) or less commonly from the blood via the kidney (descending infection). Rarely infection may extend from neighbouring structures. The transient presence of bacteria in urine without symptoms (asymptomatic bacteriuria) is common, particularly among females, due to their short urethra.

Factors that predispose to UTI are any structural or functional abnormality of the tract that can provide a foothold for multiplication of microbes, and so convert asymptomatic bacteriuria into an infection. Abnormalities may be congenital or acquired, but in the context of HAI the most important is the passage of any device through the urethra (to produce the bacteriuria) plus even minor trauma (to help to provide the foothold). A major risk factor for patients undergoing urethral instrumentation is pre-existing UTI. In the presence of infection, diagnostic cystoscopy may turn into a lethal investigation if it precipitates septicaemia. Other than in an emergency, a patient who has or might have UTI should be cystoscoped only after bacteriological examination and, if necessary, treatment. In the absence of a laboratory, the investigation is done under cover of prophylactic antimicrobials.

The types of bacteria that cause UTI are outlined in Figure 2.3 and described in more detail in Table 4.4 (below, p. 83). They vary widely with type of patient, duration of catheterization and the pattern of antimicrobial usage in the hospital concerned. Risk factors are chronic urinary problems, prolonged catheterization and treatment in a hospital where the use of antimicrobials is uncontrolled and excessive. Such patients are found to have infections due to multiply-resistant, Gram-negative rods. *Klebsiella* spp. or *P. aeruginosa* are examples. Ultimately, *Candida* spp. may be involved.

The urinary catheter is the principal cause of hospital acquired UTI. Infecting microbes gain entry to the catheterized urinary tract at the points indicated in Figure 4.1. They may be introduced mechanically at the time of catheterization when the tip of the catheter passes through the colonized part of the urethra. Later they may travel through the space between the outside of the catheter and the urethral mucosa (extraluminal spread), or enter through the lumen of the catheter itself (intraluminal spread). The presence of a catheter favours the abnormal multiplication of bacteria in the urethra. Sooner or later these bacteria reach the bladder, assisted by small reciprocal movements of the catheter generated by patient activity. The anchoring of the catheter to prevent pressure on the neck of the bladder by the self-retaining balloon helps to minimize this movement. The bacteria concerned, as well as those introduced at the time of catheterization, are likely to have originated in patients' normal flora, perhaps modified by hospital stay (Chapter 2, p. 12). Most cases of UTI are self-infections, perhaps of the autogenous type (Chapter 2, p. 29). Bacteria that gain entry by the intraluminal route are more likely to have originated on the hands of staff, and so these cases of UTI are due to cross-infection.

Once bacteria reach the bladder, they multiply and colonize the urine. This, initially, symptomless bacteriuria differs from the transient form seen in normal people because it persists as long as the catheter is in place. The free multiplication of bacteria eventually turns colonization into infection. The transition is obscured in catheterized patients because they cannot suffer from frequency and dysuria, the usual early symptoms of UTI. Perhaps only a quarter of patients with catheter-associated bacteriuria develop symptoms. It is difficult to decide which of the others are suffering from subclinical infections, and so require antimicrobial therapy. Bacteriuria nearly always resolves when the catheter is removed, and so this is the simplest form of treatment. If this is not possible, a decision to use antimicrobials will depend on risk assessment. The presence of neutropenia, or of symptoms suggesting renal involvement with the danger of septicaemia, are factors to be taken into account. Unfortunately, the usual result of treatment is to exchange the microbe initially present for one more resistant, and septicaemia sometimes complicates asymptomatic bacteriuria. The decision to withold treatment is not easily made.

Catheter-related UTI may be caused by self-infection or cross-infection. The relative importance of the two routes may be judged by noting the large difference between the rates of colonization and infection following open (100% after four days) and closed drainage (100% delayed to 30 days). Properly used, closed drainage virtually eliminates intraluminal cross-infection, but it cannot influence extraluminal self-infection. If, after catheterization, a patients' urines becomes contaminated too early, the most likely cause is failure to keep the system closed. It may be necessary to break the connection between catheter and collection system to irrigate the bladder to remove blood clots. The need to do this can be reduced if a three-way catheter is used. Note, however, that multilumen catheters make it possible to convert a closed system into an open one, unless particular care is taken. As a cardinal rule, closed systems should not be opened for trivial reasons. Urine samples should be collected from the closed system with a syringe and needle and **not** by breaking the connection between catheter and bag and, of course, never from the drainage tap.

Catheterization is usually ended after a few days, and so in most cases the bag does not need to be changed at all. In long-term catheterization, catheters should be changed as determined by patient assessment, and the collection system should be changed at the same time. The only regular reason for opening the system is to drain the urine collected in the catheter bag. Intraluminal spread of bacteria into the bladder is often preceded by colonization of this urine. This is a result of carelessness when emptying the bag. Emptying should be a careful, clean procedure. Hands should be washed before and after emptying, and a plastic apron worn if splashing is likely. The jug or vessel should be thoroughly washed and dried between each use or, better, put though the washer-disinfector used for cleaning bedpans and urinals. Gloves are only necessary if the bag used is constructed so that contamination of the hands with urine is likely. Drainage taps should be designed to prevent this. A nurse who takes a jug from bag to bag without intervening disinfection and handcare is negligent.

Strategies for preventing the entry of bacteria into the urinary tract differ according to the route they follow. Intraluminal spread is blocked most surely by keeping the system closed and taking care when emptying the bag. It has been suggested that the addition of a disinfectant to bags prevents bacterial colonization of urine, and some collecting systems are manufactured with non-return valves in them to prevent the reflux of, perhaps, infected urine into the bladder. Neither has been effective in all trials, and in any case these measures are only necessary if simple primary rules are broken. The bag should not, of course, be raised above the level of the urethra, or allowed to trail on the floor. If there is a risk of reflux (when a patient is being moved for instance), the tubing should be clamped first.

The initial entry of bacteria into the bladder is limited if meticulous attention is paid to procedure at catheter insertion. The lubrication of the urethra with an anaesthetic jelly containing an antiseptic has been shown to reduce the rate of infection. It has been suggested the use of catheters made of silicone rubber limits the development of abnormal bacterial colonization in the space between the catheter and the wall of the urethra. The same advantage may be produced if ordinary catheters are coated with materials possessing special physical or disinfectant properties. Benefits from these innovations have been hard to prove, or still await assessment. The regular use of disinfectants round the urinary meatus appeals to logic, but the results of trials conflict. The likely reason for the failure of this approach is that abnormal colonization of the urethra is most often initiated at catheter insertion. Disinfectants applied to the meatus do not reach the whole length of the urethra, which cannot be sterilized prior to catheterization. While catheters are in place, washing of the perineal area to a good standard of personal hygiene is sufficient. With non-ambulant patients, perineal care with soap and water at a frequency determined by nursing assessment is substituted.

Long-term catheterization in patients with spinal injury due to trauma or disease is always associated with bacteriuria and UTI. This is a major cause of mortality in these cases. Attempts at control is a specialized subject with a large literature to which reference should be made by those concerned with the problem.

The incidence of hospital acquired UTI can be reduced by avoiding catheterization whenever possible and by removing catheters at the earliest possible moment. Those who catheterize for convenience should be reminded that catheter insertion carries a mortality. A catheter should **never** be used just to collect a specimen of urine. If catheters were available only on prescription, their use would diminish. Incontinence pads can replace some catheterization with benefit to infection rates, but their use is associated with disposal problems. The use of condom-like collection systems for males reduce infections, but care is needed to avoid damage to the skin of the penis. Suprapubic drainage reduces the chances of infection by the urethral route, but is perhaps too invasive for short-term use. Intermittent catheterization might replace both short- and long-term catheterization. In good hands, this reduces infections, but care is necessary to avoid trauma to the urethra.

It should be possible to monitor colonizations or infections in catheterized patients and react appropriately if they are too high. This will involve some routine culture of urine, though general bacteriological testing is not cost effective. A sampling system should be devised, concentrating on departments of the hospital where the rates of UTI are higher (Figure 2.2). As with all such surveys, the active involvement of the clinical staff helps to ensure that the survey is properly performed, and that the findings are acted upon.

WOUND INFECTIONS

A wound has been defined as an injury to the body caused by physical means with disruption of the normal continuity of body structures. In this broad sense, a wound may result from any accidental or deliberate trauma that breaks the surface of skin or mucous membrane. Pressure sores and ulcers due to vascular or neural pathology may be included. The points of entry of tubes or wires into body cavities or the cardio-vascular system are also wounds. As these are considered below (p. 79) and in Chapter 5 (p. 91), they are not dealt with here.

Using the broad definition given, we are concerned with accidental wounds, burns, surgical wounds, ulcers and pressure sores. Accidental wounds, usually, and burns are often subject to surgery, so join opera-tive wounds as 'surgical'. To lump them together may seem harmless, but it has, in fact, led to the inappropriate and expensive extension of practices that might be applicable to one kind of wound to the treat-ment of other kinds (Colebrook *et al.*, 1948). In the context of HAI, it is important to distinguish between wounds in which subcutaneous tissues are exposed to the outside world for days or weeks, and those where the exposure is limited to minutes or hours. In the first category are burns, pressure sores, traumatic or other wounds with loss of superficial tissue, and surgical wounds resulting from the treatment of missile or blast injuries in which skin closure is postponed (delayed primary suture). In the second category are the wounds that arise from the great mass of elective and acute surgical operations.

Haemolytic streptococcal infections of burns and of the wartime wounds treated by delayed primary suture were the subject of intense study in the 1940s. With large areas of more or less devitalized tissue exposed for long periods, these wounds were perfect culture media for haemolytic streptococci, which were the most feared of hospital pathogens at the time. Colonization, infection and, in some cases, septicaemia tended to follow in a progression. Once introduced into a unit, cross-infection ensured that each wound quickly became home to an enormous population of streptococci. From there they were available to contaminate the hands of staff and the environment, and so a vicious circle was created. In these circumstances, it was a matter of observation that wartime surgical wounds became infected postoperatively, in the ward (Miles, 1944). In the case of burns, inves-tigators felt that infection was being transmitted through the air as well as by physical contact with members of staff. Filtration of the air was introduced to control the airborne route, and the 'no-touch' dressing technique was employed to control contact spread (Colebrook, 1955). Quantities of disinfectants were used to decontaminate the environment.

In a situation like this, why does simple handwashing, perhaps with a disinfectant, not work as it had for Semmelweis (Chapter 1)? The answer is that streptococci reach, by touch or by falling out of the air, a devitalized surface lacking normal defences including polymorphonuclear leucocytes (Chapter 2, p. 35), so that it resembles a permanently open Petri dish of blood agar already at the ideal temperature of a bacteriological incubator. In these circumstances, even cocci that have already lost their infectivity due to drying and even too few in number to get a foothold in a normal person are able to multiply to produce a colonization. This soon becomes an infection as the colonizers grow into a large population of now fully virulent streptococci. The uterine wounds of Semmelweis' patients were poorly accessible to airborne microbes and did not lack PML. His success was immediate when he dealt with the hands that were the main vector of fresh, fully virulent streptococci. What is true for streptococci is in general also true for staphylococci or other bacterial pathogens. This explains why even the most elaborate care cannot prevent colonization of wounds in a burns unit, where infections are so common. These units will be considered further in Chapter 6 (p. 140). Burns, wounds treated by delayed primary suture where debridement has been inadequate and pressure sores are all special cases. When wounds of these types are concentrated in a ward or unit, they tend to be colonized or infected by indistinguishable (so probably identical) bacteria as a result of cross-infection, or even by environmental infection that is unimportant in other areas.

None of this is true of ordinary surgical wounds, where tissues are exposed to the outside world only briefly, and where innate immunity still functions. Infection of these wounds is much less common, and even in the same unit at the same time the bacteria that cause them are often different. Infected surgical wounds are typically distributed in a hospital as shown in Figure 2.2, and the bacteria characteristically involved are outlined in Figure 2.3 and given in greater detail in Table 4.4, p. 83. The single most common pathogen in surgical wound infection (SWI) is *Staph. aureus*. In NUH, this was involved in 40% of SWI, divided between ordinary strains in 22% and MARSA in 18%. A variety of GNRs were responsible in 36% of cases.

As with any infection (Chapter 2, p. 9) a complex 'soil and seed' relationship exists between the patient's tissues and colonizing bacteria. At the end of an operation, all surgical wounds contain some bacteria. When the wound is closed, the question is if these contaminating colonists can overcome the local defences and establish an infection. The outcome turns on the balance between host resistance on one hand, and bacterial numbers and virulence on the other. The number of bacteria that can be dealt with by local defences is very large (Chapter 2, p. 12), but this ability may be compromised by a number of factors, summarized in Table 4.1.

The local factors listed under (1) in Table 4.1 are to a large extent under the direct control of the surgeon. Hippocrates recommended

Table 4.1 The factors on the patient's side that influence the development of a surgical wound infection

---

The soil
Subcutaneous tissue exposed through a wound at operation
fertilized by:

1. local factors,
       dead tissue, haematomas
       poor circulation, foreign bodies
2. general factors,
       patient debility (age, obesity, illness)
       immune deficiency

– as may be modified by prophylactic antimicrobials.

---

that wounds be treated gently and, at the beginning of the modern era of surgery, Halsted propounded the basic principles of wound care. Evidence to be produced later shows that surgeons sometimes need to be reminded that complete haemostasis, preservation of a sufficient blood supply, removal of devitalized tissue, obliteration of dead space, and wound closure without tension are important if infections are to be avoided. Foreign bodies in a wound reduce by a large factor the number of bacteria that can be handled by tissue defences (Chapter 2, p. 12). Sutures, ligatures and tissue killed by diathermy have been joined by a growing list of novel foreign bodies, such as spare parts made of plastic, metal or animal tissues.

In an emergency, there may be no time to do anything about the general factors (Table 4.1) that make the soil of wounds more fertile for the bacterial seed. Infections already present can be treated and diabetes controlled. If the circumstances allow, elective surgery may be delayed until obesity or malnutrition have been dealt with. The effect of antimicrobial prophylaxis may be profound, but this should not be used to hide surgical inadequacy.

Having examined the factors that may alter the susceptibility of a wound to infection, the microbial components of the equation require attention. If logic is to be applied to the prevention of SWI, it is necessary to analyse the sources and vectors (Chapter 2, p. 28) of the pathogens concerned. The possible sources are shown in Table 4.2. The most common pathogen, *Staph. aureus*, may be found as part of the normal flora of the skin. Thus it may originate in the patient, his or her attendants, or in a part of the environment previously contaminated by

Table 4.2 The possible sources of the bacteria that might cause surgical wound infections

---

The seed
Microbial contamination of a wound arising from:

1. patients'
    skin
    colonized hollow organs
    abnormal colonizations or infections
 – arising by direct extension into the wound or through the blood, at the time of operation or later
2. staff, before, during or after operation
3. the environment, before, during or after operation.

---

a carrier, and so all three routes of infection are possibilities. These can be narrowed down most effectively by examining the incidence of SWI after different operative procedures.

It is customary to divide operations into four or more classes, each associated with a different risk of infection (Appendix, p. 169). In a series of over 60 000 studied by the Canadian surgeon Peter Cruse, clean operations were associated with a rate of SWI of 1.5%. The figure for clean-contaminated operations was 7.7%, and contaminated and dirty operations had SWI rates of 15.2 and 40.0%, respectively (Cruse, 1986). In other studies in which operations were categorized in this way, similarly graded rates of infection have been noted. The point about Cruse' study was that patients were allocated randomly among a group of operating rooms, and postoperatively they were distributed again at random to a set of surgical wards. In this way, patients were treated similarly with respect to exposure of their wounds to environmental infection and, with the exception of the surgeon, to the risks of cross-infection as well. How may the large differences in the incidence of infection between clean and the other classes of surgery be accounted for?

When examined in detail, the results showed that the rates of infection were the same for each operating room and ward. As just noted, rates varied according to the class of operation, but they also differed between surgeons. This difference was much more dramatic when clean surgery only was considered and the different types of surgery (general, orthopaedic, etc.) were separated. It was found that some surgeons were regularly returning rates of SWI following clean operations three or more times that of the 'best' of their colleagues. This was true for all the types of surgery. The inevitable conclusion was that environmental infection and cross-infection from OR and ward staff (excluding the surgeon who operated) was responsible for no more than the lowest rate of infection scored by the 'best' surgeon. A further conclusion was that the contribution of postoperative care to SWI in clean wounds was negligible. This is not surprising because the skin edges of a wound closed at the end of an operation seal together sufficiently within a few hours to prevent the entry of bacteria. Drainage by **closed** vacuum methods does not alter this. The observation that wounds do not get infected in the ward allowed the hospital to save money by simplifying postoperative wound care.

The statement that surgical wounds are impervious to the entry of bacteria after a few hours requires some expansion. Biological functions rarely have definable points at which something is untrue at one moment and true the next. Even death defies definition in such simple terms, and so it is with surgical wounds. The reason is explained in physiology textbooks where blood clotting, the starting point for wound healing, is described. In this case, the process is taking place in the insensible gap between the opposing surfaces of the wound. A cascade of events follow one another to convert soluble fibrinogen to fibrin, an insoluble polymer that is laid down initially as a loose, weak mesh. This happens within minutes, and in the following few hours this loose network consolidates and contracts to form a much firmer structure into which fibroblasts begin to grow, laying down collagen as a prelude to final healing. Provided the wound is not forcibly torn apart, this progression renders a wound increasingly impervious to the entry of bacteria from the outside at a rate that proceeds most rapidly at the outset and gets slower as time passes. There is no point at which a wound suddenly becomes impervious to anything, but the process is substantially complete once the clot has retracted and has been anchored in place by the first fibroblasts. The speed with which this happens varies according to circumstances, but in nearly every case 'within a few hours' is a fair estimate.

Once Cruse had largely eliminated general cross-infection and environmental infection as the causes of surgical wound infections, there remained either the patient or his or her surgeon as sources of the microbes that caused it. If the patient was the source, then the best point at which to reduce the risk may be assessed from Table 4.1. The factor most readily modified is (1), surgical technique. When he found large and significant differences in infection rates between surgeons, Cruse informed them individually of their sepsis rates, with the performance of the others (given anonymously) for comparison. There was an immediate and dramatic improvement, and the **overall** sepsis rate in clean surgery was halved. In this way, surgeons were ruled out as important sources of the **microbes** that caused the infections, though they were revealed as the **causes** of most of them. Self-infection was left as the dominant source of the microbes that cause SWI. These findings have been confirmed independently in a more recent study (Mishriki *et al.*, 1990). It appears that the contribution of some surgeons to SWI is inadvertently to add to the fertility of the soil rather than to supply the seed.

Other important conclusions emerged from Cruse' study. Several of these reconfirmed observations previously made by others. The longer a patient stayed in hospital preoperatively, the greater the chance of postoperative wound infection. The use of adhesive plastic drapes was associated with a higher rate of sepsis than the use of waterproof or water-repellent disposable or reusable ones. Skin disinfection was best done with an active antiseptic with a residual action; in Cruse' study this was used in conjunction with alcohol. Alcohol is an excellent, fast-acting disinfectant. It does not need nor should it be applied in such quantities as to leave pools of flammable liquid that might be ignited by electrodiathermy. Shaving the operative site with a sharp razor was found to be contraindicated; the use of electric clippers was associated with a lower rate of SWI, and a depilatory cream (or no shaving at all) produced the lowest rate. In fact, there is no **microbiological** reason for preoperative shaving (Chapter 2, p. 31). Removal of hair in the immediate locality may be desirable to keep it out of the operative field, and allow adhesive dressings to stick to the skin.

Over 10% of pairs of gloves were found to be punctured post-operatively. Perhaps because surgeons 'scrubbed' with an antiseptic detergent having a residual action (chlorhexidine), none of the patients apparently exposed to risk due to these punctures developed wound infections as a result. 'Scrubbing' with a brush was usually limited to the first case in a list. The study confirmed once more that without a 28-day follow up, a significant number of SWIs are missed. With hospital stay getting progressively shorter, the follow-up of patients into the community is essential for accurate surveillance of surgical sepsis. Without it, the shortfall may exceed 20%.

Quantitative ideas help to understand these findings. A study found that over half the wounds that contain more than 100 000 bacteria per gram of tissue at the time of closure became infected afterwards. Wounds containing less than this number of bacteria healed without infection (Krizek and Robson, 1975). Body defences can overcome a large bacterial challenge. The number of bacteria on or in healthy skin varies, but an upper figure of 400 000 per cm^2 has been recorded (Chapter 2, p. 30). About 20% of skin bacteria remain alive after effective surgical disinfection, and so this figure may be reduced to a maximum of 80 000 at the beginning of surgery. The bacteria concerned will usually be members of the normal skin flora, perhaps modified by stay in hospital (Chapter 2, p. 12). *Staph. epidermidis* is, therefore, one of the less pathogenic though more universal contaminants. A proportion of people are carriers of the much more pathogenic *Staph. aureus* (Chapter 2, p. 30). When found on the skin, they are usually present in hair follicles, just below the skin surface. Here they are secure from the effects of shaving and are protected from disinfectants. It is easy to imagine that in such people the number of *Staph. aureus* in a wound may multiply to exceed the watershed figure of 100 000 per gram of tissue before it is closed.

This is particularly true when the patient has been shaved pre-operatively. Shaving inevitably causes minor abrasions in which any *Staph. aureus* present will start to multiply, their number increasing as the gap widens between the time of shaving and the beginning of the operation. Of course, if the wound involves a contaminated hollow viscus, such as the gut, the number of microbes needed to initiate an infection is likely to be exceeded manyfold, and the bacterial species concerned are more likely to be GNRs or anaerobes. In elective operations involving the colon, preoperative preparation of the bowel is designed to reduce the level of this contamination. Surgical invasion of such sites explains why clean-contaminated and contaminated operations have higher rates of infection than clean ones. These numerical considerations support the idea that most SWI is self-infection.

Alternative sources of the microbes that cause SWI are the OR staff and the environment. It has already been noted that these can only cause something less than the lowest rate of SWI achieved in clean surgery. Staff carry bacteria in the same way as patients but, given even elementary care, it is difficult to imagine a route by which the number of bacteria necessary to cause an infection might be transferred to a wound. Even a glove puncture is unlikely to leak the large number required, particularly if an antiseptic surgical scrub with a residual action has been used.

There remains the environment. Bacteria that settle on inanimate surfaces usually adhere to them firmly, so unless the surface itself is put into a wound, they are harmless. Bacteria suspended in the air are different, as they might fall into a wound, or on to exposed instruments or other items that are to be put into it. The only important source of bacteria found in the air of an OR are the bodies of its occupants (Chapter 2, p. 30). In a badly ventilated OR, these might reach a count of 20 bacteria-carrying particles (mainly skin squames) per cubic foot (706 per m^3). Particles fall out of the air at a rate depending on their size, but in a bad OR, about 100 average-sized, bacteria-carrying particles would settle every hour on an open wound measuring $10\,in^2$ ($65\,cm^2$). Even though many particles carry more than one bacterium, most are of less pathogenic species, *Staph. epidermidis*, for instance. It is difficult to imagine airborne microbes reaching the critical level of 100 000 per gram during ordinary operating, even when those falling on to instruments are added. The numerical difference between the potential for causing SWI by self-infection and by cross- or environmental infection is very large.

It is necessary to remember that cross- and environmental infections are closely connected in ORs, as the microbes concerned both come from the same place. Effectively, all airborne bacteria in an OR and by extension those on inanimate surfaces are derived from the bodies and, principally, the skin of its occupants (Chapter 2, p. 30). The suits of woven fabric usually worn in ORs are not a barrier to the passage of microbes from the skin. This is due to their style with openings at various points and, particularly, to the material from which they are made. Fabric so closely woven as to be impervious to skin squames and the bacteria they carry is uncomfortable to wear, as it also limits the passage of perspiration.

What has been said applies to the great mass of general surgery, in which infections, though regrettable and costly, do not often seriously prejudice a successful outcome. The outlook is good in clean surgery where, with care, infection rates as low as 1–2% are achievable. The higher rates of sepsis in other classes of surgery are improving with the help of carefully designed antimicrobial prophylaxis. However, as modern surgery becomes more complex, and particularly where foreign materials are implanted in critical sites, even a 1–2% rate of infection is too much. An infection that loosens a hip replacement is a tragedy; an infection round a prosthetic heart valve may be lethal. In cases like this, there is a strong stimulus to assess the real contribution to surgical sepsis of the cross- and environmental routes of infection to see if already low rates can be made even lower.

Although it dates back to 1959, the US National Research Council study of the effect of irradiating the air in ORs with ultraviolet (uV) light provides relevant information (National Research Council, 1964). In this study, nearly 15 000 patients were operated on in ORs fitted with uV lamps designed to irradiate the air to kill airborne bacteria. Each OR had two lamps, one real, the other a dummy that emitted a blue light, and so staff did not know one from the other. These lamps were switched on alternately in a predetermined way. Operative procedures were classified according to the risk of infection, using five categories rather than the four employed by Cruse. The effect of the uV light was to reduce the count of airborne bacteria by 50–60%. Overall infection rates were 7.4% for operations done under uV, and 7.5% when the dummy lamps were on. Only in the refined clean class (elective clean operations closed without drainage) was a significant difference noted: 2.9% infections under uV compared with 3.8% without.

A more recent study was conducted in the UK by the Medical Research Council (Lidwell *et al.*, 1982). This involved just over 8000 operations for the implantation of hip or knee prostheses. These were done in conventional ORs or in ORs with ultra-clean air (laminar flow) ventilation. During some of the operations in the latter, additional all-enveloping, impermeable, exhaust-ventilated suits were worn by the operating team. These special measures reduced the number of airborne microbes by between 70% and 99%. Unfortunately, the use of antimicrobial prophylaxis was not controlled in the trial. Deep surgical wound infections were recorded in 3.4% of patients who did not receive antimicrobial prophylaxis and who were operated on in conventional ORs. When operations were done under ultra-clean conditions this rate was halved, and the rate was halved again (to 0.9%) when exhaust suits were used. Prophylactic antimicrobials on their own reduced the deep sepsis rate to 0.8%. Retrospective attempts were made by the investigators to untangle the effects of antimicrobials and clean air by excluding some contributors. With this selective approach, the interpretation most favourable to ultra-clean air was that when combined with prophylaxis (without exhaust suits), there were 43 fewer cases of deep sepsis for each 10 000 operations done compared with operations performed in conventional ORs under prophylaxis. The interpretation using all the data without any retrospective exclusion is that there would have been 11 fewer cases (Meers 1983a, b).

Different positions are taken about the cost effectiveness of providing the extra facilities necessary to produce improvements of this order, and what those facilities should be. The conclusion is that in operations where relatively large areas of tissue are exposed for longer periods and foreign bodies are implanted, some airborne infection does take place, but that much of it may be prevented by antimicrobial prophylaxis. It is evident that something about these implant operations reduces the number of bacteria needed to initiate an infection compared with non-prosthetic surgery. It is not clear if the foreign body on its own is a sufficient cause. It would be a very expensive mistake to allow this limited conclusion to influence practice in general surgery. Because most operations are completed more quickly, with less exposed tissue and the addition of little extraneous foreign material, the small contribution the air makes to infection in prosthetic

surgery becomes largely irrelevant by comparison with the higher
infection rates experienced in general surgery.

It is a pity that the MRC trial did not include a group operated on in
conventional ORs by surgical teams wearing exhaust suits. As the
source of airborne bacteria in ORs is the human body, it may be
that wearing these suits removes the need for ultra-clean air. In this
context, it is notable that the head is one of the more heavily bacterially
colonized areas of the skin. It has been shown that the rubbing of
masks increases the shedding of bacteria from the face (Schweizer,
1976), and so it is likely that caps and the necklines of gowns do the
same. Any larger particles rubbed off in this way from the faces and
necks of surgeons and assistants are more likely to fall directly into the
sterile field. This short and direct airborne route of infection can only
be blocked by wearing full exhaust suits, though it might be less
important if masks were not worn (Chapter 5, p. 102).

It is increasingly difficult to make further properly controlled
advances in the prevention of SWI. It can be deduced from Figure 2.6
that control and test groups of prohibitive size would be required in a
trial designed to detect a 25% improvement in a sepsis rate already
as low as 1.5%. In fact, the figure approaches 20 000, or a total of 40 000
operations. A multicentre trial involving so many surgeons would be
needed that it would almost certainly fail under the weight of its own
complexity. In these circumstances, it is tempting to make deductions
from experiments in which microbes are pursued in and out of the
environment with no connection made to infections. The history of
infection control shows that this approach leads to expensive errors.

RESPIRATORY TRACT INFECTIONS

The respiratory tract is divided into two by the larynx. The upper part
starts at the nostrils, where inspired air passes into the nasal cavity and
backwards into the nasopharynx. Air then travels through the oral and
laryngeal pharynx. These parts of the respiratory tract are shared with
the alimentary canal. Next it enters the lower respiratory tract through
the vocal cords in the larynx. Passing through the trachea, bronchi and
bronchioles it eventually reaches the alveoli.

Apart from the front of the nasal cavity and the part shared with the
alimentary canal and the alveoli themselves, the respiratory tract is
lined with a ciliated columnar epithelium. It is, therefore, covered by a
mass of microscopic hair-like cilia that are in constant motion. Scattered
among the epithelial cells are mucus secreting cells that produce a
carpet of sticky mucus on the top of the cilia. The cilia beat to and fro,

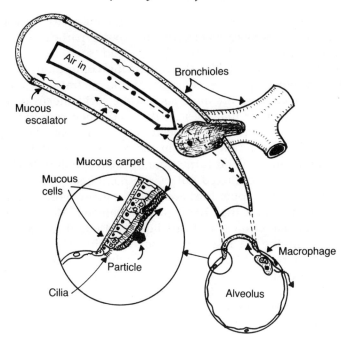

Figure 4.2 The principal natural defence mechanisms of the lower respiratory tract, with particles trapped by the mucous carpet and removed by the mucous escalator, or dealt with by alveolar macrophages.

strongly in one direction, and limply in the other. This keeps the mucus in motion, and as the cilia are co-ordinated, the movement of the mucus is one-way. The direction is upwards towards the larynx in the lower part of the tract, and downwards from the other. Mucus on this 'mucous escalator' arrives in the oral or laryngeal part of the pharynx, where it is usually swallowed, or it may be expectorated (Figure 4.2).

It is often said that the function of the lining of the respiratory tract is to warm and humidify the inspired air. This is true, but it has a third and very vital function. It helps to keep the lower tract (and some parts of the upper) free of microbes, so making them into the privileged surfaces described in Chapter 2 (p. 11) and Figure 2.1.

The air contains enormous numbers of tiny particles. A variable but small proportion of these carry microbes (mostly bacteria, viruses and fungal spores). With the exception of fungal spores, it is unusual for microbes to travel on their own. One or more of them are carried on a raft or inside a fragment of other material (Chapter 2, p. 30). The effect of this is that most particles that carry microbes are very much bigger than the microbes themselves. If airborne particles were inhaled unchecked, the respiratory passages would soon be clogged, and infection would be inevitable. The combination of tortuous air passages and the mucous carpet prevent this. As the air travels round bends, the particles it contains are flung against the sticky mucus on the walls of the tract, like a car that goes off the road when cornering too fast. Depending on the site above or below the larynx, particles trapped in this way are swept down or up on the mucous escalator at a rate of about 16 mm a minute and carried out of the respiratory tract.

Large particles are filtered out by the hairs inside the nostrils. The mucus carpet of the upper tract accounts for many more, and nearly all those measuring more than 10 microns in diameter. Most of the smaller ones (and the larger ones as well when breathing through the mouth) are caught in the trachea and upper bronchi. Smaller and lighter particles more readily 'take the bends': a light sports car can go round a corner more easily than a heavy lorry. More and more of the smaller particles are trapped as the air containing them travels down the bronchi and bronchioles. To reach the alveoli, a particle must be smaller than 5 microns, and ideally 1–2 microns in diameter. Particles that penetrate this far meet a new defender, the macrophage. These phagocytic cells engulf small particles and then remove them by crawling out of the alveolus to mount the mucous escalator, or by entering the lymphatic system. Particles smaller than 1 micron tend to make the round trip without striking any surface, and are exhaled (Figure 4.2).

The respiratory tract has other defence mechanisms. The cough reflex is stimulated by larger particles landing in the larynx, trachea and larger bronchi. A variety of chemical and cellular elements of both the innate and adaptive immune systems (Chapter 2, p. 11) also operate in the respiratory tract.

The defences that protect the lower respiratory tract may be compromised in various ways. Sometimes cilia are congenitally ineffective. Their activity is suppressed by tobacco smoke, alcohol, the misuse of drugs or by infections. Some viruses and mycoplasmas are particularly harmful as they destroy the ciliated epithelium. This also happens in whooping cough. Toxic agents may inhibit the cough reflex. As contributors to HAI, the factors listed are joined by some therapeutic drugs, particularly of the morphine group and the anaesthetic agents. Tracheal intubation (either for anaesthesia or for long-term mechanical respiratory support) bypasses the principal defence by interrupting the 'up' mucous escalator. This leads to an accumulation of mucus plus any particles trapped in it that can no longer reach the pharynx.

This has to be sucked out mechanically, offering an opportunity for cross-infection. Heavily contaminated secretions also collect above the balloon on the endotracheal tube, perhaps to leak past it, and certainly to run down into the lower tract when it is deflated.

Infections of the respiratory tract (like its anatomy) are divided into upper and lower. Infections may commence in the upper respiratory tract and stay there, descend from upper to lower, or begin as lower respiratory infections (LRI). Infections of the upper tract may be trivial (a light cold) or very unpleasant (acute sinusitis), but do not often threaten the lives of healthy people. Many are caused by viruses. Some of these, including the respiratory syncytial virus and influenza viruses, may cause life-threatening descending infections in infancy and old age respectively, and these may be hospital acquired. Cases of hospital acquired LRI are more serious, and if pneumonia and septicaemia develop, may be lethal. Infection of the upper tract is not a notable feature of HAI, but bacterial pneumonia is an important component of it. To what extent LRI is secondary to preliminary viral infections is not known. The frequency and distribution of LRI in hospitals is described in Chapter 2, pp. 17 and 18, and in Figure 2.2. The latter illustrates the concentration of these infections in all six ICUs, with a lower but still significant incidence in surgical and medical wards. In the latter, they are associated with breathing difficulties after abdominal operations or the admission to medical wards of patients predisposed to infection because they are suffering from organic lung disease or the results of a cerebrovascular accident.

A summary of the microbial causes of LRI is given in Figure 2.3, with more detail in Table 4.4, p. 83. In general, GNRs are the most frequent causes of hospital acquired LRI. This was the case in NUH between 1986 and 1989 (44% of all LRI were due to GNRs among which *P. aeruginosa* caused 19%, *Klebsiella* spp. 12% and others 14%). *Staph. aureus* was next most frequent (33%), divided between 'ordinary' strains 8% and MARSA 25%. Other bacteria were the cause in 23% of cases. Other centres have recorded a higher incidence of infections due to GNRs than was noted in NUH, ranging up to 60%.

The chain of events that leads to hospital acquired LRI due to GNRs is well known. GNRs rarely reside in a healthy pharynx, but they are commonly found there in seriously ill patients. It seems this is due at least in part to the loss of an important surface component of oropharyngeal cells called fibronectin. When present, this material encourages the adhesion of Gram-positive bacterial cells. In its absence, GNRs adhere freely. The saliva of seriously ill patients is likely to contain an enzyme that destroys fibronectin. They are also more likely to be treated with antimicrobials. Their disordered normal oropharyngeal flora almost certainly includes multi-resistant GNRs. The breakdown of respiratory defences allows these GNRs to enter, colonize and, perhaps, infect the lower respiratory tract. Tracheal intubation for mechanical ventilation is an excellent way of achieving this breakdown, and this is why LRI is so common in ICUs (Figure 2.2). In hospitals, this is where serious debility, extensive antimicrobial therapy and assisted respiration are most likely to coexist. It follows that LRI due to GNRs is most often a self-infection of the autogenous kind (Figure 2.4). Cross-infection also plays a part because tracheal tubes are subjected to a lot of handling.

Staphylococcal LRI may develop similarly. In NUH, MARSA was found more often than more sensitive staphylococci as the cause of this, so cross-infection may play a part. Where there is a tracheostomy, there is a wound which, like any other wound, may be the site of a staphylococcal infection (above, p. 66). This is another source of bacteria that may be introduced into the respiratory tract when the tracheostomy tube is manipulated. This is probably why infections are more common in patients ventilated through a tracheostomy than when other routes are used.

The other potential source of infecting microbes is the environment, in particular, ventilators. Humidification of inspired air is now more often done with a humidifier rather than a nebulizer, which reduces the chances that contaminated water is sprayed into the patient. However, any wet environment is a potential hazard (Chapter 2, p. 37), and this one requires special attention. Humidification of the inspired air and condensation of water from the expired air make ventilator tubing wet, and so support the growth of GNRs. This tubing requires to be changed at intervals. This should be done carefully, as a clean procedure, the hands being washed before and after each change. Opinions vary on the frequency of these changes, and although the decision is somewhat arbitrary, it has financial consequences. A change every 24 hours was commonly recommended, but recently authoratative sources have suggested that they may be used safely for 48 hours. Changes may be made less frequently if heat-moisture exchangers are used, and sometimes in neonates (Cadwallader *et al.*, 1990).

Other risk factors associated with a higher incidence of RTI are age, immunosuppression and surgery. Each time the endotracheal balloon is deflated, heavily contaminated secretions trapped above it slide into the lower part of the tract where the interrupted mucous escalator cannot remove them. Another risk factor is the use of cimetidine or ranitidine to suppress gastric acidity to prevent the development of stress ulcers and gastrointestinal bleeding. Gastric acidity is the normal defence mechanism that keeps the stomach almost free of bacteria and protects the intestines from invasion by organisms present in food. In the absence of acid, the stomach is colonized by a variety of bacteria that may regurgitate through the oesophagus into the pharynx and so reach the larynx. This is particularly likely if a nasogastric tube is in place. The use of sucralfate has been recommended, as this protects the gastrointestinal mucosa from injury without inhibiting or neutralizing gastric acid.

The diagnosis of hospital acquired RTI is often difficult. The progression over a period perhaps measured in days from a colonization of the trachea by potentially pathogenic bacteria to tracheobronchitis to pneumonia means that bacteriological criteria on their own are of no use. The development of a cough or the new production of sputum normally useful in clinical diagnosis do not apply in an intubated patient, who may also be febrile or have a raised white cell count for other reasons. X-rays may not help. Post-mortem studies have shown that ante-mortem diagnosis of this form of HAI is very unreliable. The problem is that the best diagnostic methods (transtracheal aspiration, bronchoscopic examination, needle or open biopsy) either cannot be applied to patients attached to mechanical ventilators, or they have an unacceptably high morbidity in seriously ill patients, or both.

OTHER INFECTIONS

The 'other' infections are those left when the three more common ones (UTI, SWI and LRI) are removed. Their numbers and types vary from survey to survey, depending on the definitions used, the mixture of patients in the hospitals concerned, and whether or not such things as mild upper respiratory infections are included. Table 2.2 shows that in 12 large surveys, 'other' infections averaged 23% of all HAI. This figure is quite close to the 20% found in NUH between 1986 and 1989 (Table 2.2). Although these infections vary between surveys, those found in NUH (Chapter 2, p. 18) are presented for illustrative purposes. Table 4.3 compares the incidence of the more numerous 'other' infections with the more common varieties. They will be discussed in order of their frequency.

Infections associated with intravascular cannulae

Patients' cardiovascular systems are invaded with great frequency for diagnostic or therapeutic purposes. Here we are concerned only with cannulation, procedures that involve the placement of metal or plastic

Table 4.3 Incidence of different forms of HAI per 1000 cases in NUH Singapore, 1986–9

Rate/1000 cases of HAI	
UTI	412
SWI	255
LRI	133
'Other' infections:	
ICI	60
Septicaemia	42
Skin	28
GI	11
Pressure sore	5
All others	54

Key: urinary tract infection; SWI, surgical wound infection; LRI, lower respiratory infection; ICI, intravascular cannula-associated infection; GI, gastrointestinal infection.

tubes into veins or arteries for periods varying from an hour to weeks or months. In some countries, more than half of all hospital patients are cannulated.

The tubes involved are peripheral or central venous catheters, including steel needles, cuffed catheters for long-term use, catheters for the delivery of total parenteral nutrition (TPN), balloon-tipped catheters used for sampling and monitoring in the central pulmonary circulation and arterial and umbilical catheters. They are all subject to the same problems of infection, but suffer to a greater or lesser extent depending on their thickness, the length of the intravascular portion, the material from which they are made and the chemical nature of the material, if any, being infused, and the length of time they are left in place. Cannulas inserted through areas of skin with a more abundant normal flora, such as the lower limb (particularly in the groin) or into the umbilicus, are more likely to be associated with an infection than those inserted at other sites.

Vascular cannulation offers a highroad for bacteria to enter the cardiovascular system. Children and younger adults who are not severely immunocompromised can overcome a surprisingly large bacterial challenge by this route, but this ability is diminished in infants, the elderly and the immunocompromised. As with urinary catheters (above, p. 61), and endotracheal tubes (above, p. 78), bacteria gain access to the vascular system by two routes: intraluminal and extra-luminal (Chapter 5, p. 91).

Intraluminal contamination happens when microbes gain access to fluid before or during infusion or transfusion, or are present in the fluid in pressure-monitoring devices. This may happen from a variety of causes, ranging from failure during manufacture, the puncturing or cracking of containers of infusion fluids, accidents in making additions to infusions in the hospital pharmacy, ward or department, to con-tamination gaining access through the various joints in, or the supple-mentary injection ports of, giving sets, or following the attachment of piggy-back containers. Bacteria can multiply in most infusion fluids. The number of bacteria that gain access initially is usually small and unimportant, but given time a trivial contamination may turn into a lethal one. The longer the interval between contamination and infusion, the greater the danger. There have been a number of well-publicized incidents in which manufacturing failures have led months later to the use of numbers of containers of contaminated fluid, with tragic consequences (Anon, 1974). Contamination nearer the time of infusion usually involves single containers, and the hands of staff are likely to be the source of it. The sporadic cases of septicaemia that result are unlikely to be correctly attributed. They would be classified as environmental infections.

An extraluminal infection is due either to self- or cross-infection. Cannulae are inserted through skin or an umbilical stump; neither can be sterilized. Introduction is commonly percutaneous, or it may be by surgical cut-down. Unless gloves are worn, the equally unsterilizable hands of the operator making the insertion may be a source of con-tamination. Other sources are hands that manipulate the infusion apparatus later or, worse, fiddle with it unnecessarily. After a cannula has been inserted, the outer surface of its intravascular portion is likely to develop a coating of fibrin, forming a sheath one end of which is in contact with extravascular tissues at the site of skin puncture. Bacteria from the patient's skin, or the hands of a member of staff, colonize the puncture site. This process is abetted by the inevitable foreign body and the nutritious moisture that oozes from the puncture wound. In time this colonization may become an infection but, in either case, the bacteria responsible may spread down round the cannula to reach the intravascular portion. Here they may multiply protected from the body's defences. Some of these bacteria also adhere strongly to the material of which the cannula is made. When sufficient multiplication has taken place beneath the fibrin sheath, bacteria reach the surface to promote further fibrin deposition and eventually to be shed into the blood stream as infected emboli. The longer the intravascular part of the cannula, the greater the hazard. If the end of a colonized cannula lies close to or in the heart, endocardial or valvular damage and infection may develop.

As with urinary catheters (above, p. 63) adhesion of either fibrin or bacteria may be less of a problem when new more sophisticated materials are used to make intravascular cannulas. Over the years, the diameters of cannulas have been reduced, and so they present a smaller surface area for these undesirable changes. Steel needles are short and less likely to encourage adhesion of fibrin or bacteria, and so these older alternatives to plastic cannulae are safer for short-term infusions in peripheral veins. Unfortunately, if they are not inserted skilfully, their use may be complicated by extravasation of the infusion fluid into perivascular tissues.

Inflammation of a vein is phlebitis. As with any inflammation, this may be due to physical or chemical trauma as well as to infection. The physical trauma of skilful venipuncture is negligible, but inexpert puncture is not and, in any case, the long-term presence of a foreign body in a blood vessel inevitably causes some damage. Many of the fluids infused through cannulas also damage the lining of blood vessels. Some drugs given intravenously are so irritant that they must be diluted before infusion. Solutions for TPN are very corrosive and cannot be diluted sufficiently to allow them to be given into a peripheral vein. To overcome this, they are administered directly into a central vein where they are diluted directly into a large volume of rapidly flowing blood. At first, the inflammatory changes of cannula-related phlebitis may be due to non-infectious trauma. Bacteria colonizing the cannula track quickly turn this sterile inflammation into an infection. As with other forms of HAI, the precise point at which a colonization becomes an infection cannot be determined. In its ultimate state, an infectious phlebitis converts a vein into an intravascular abscess. This is rare, difficult to diagnose and potentially lethal. A patient with a persistent septicaemia who fails to respond to apparently adequate antimicrobial treatment may be suffering from suppurative phlebitis. This is a special problem with burns patients.

Authorities agree that most cannula-related sepsis is of the sporadic extraluminal type. Uncommon intraluminal infections due to the infusion of fluid contaminated at source appear as clusters of septicaemias involving the same, perhaps unusual, pathogen. Device-related infections (like their counterparts in catheter-related UTI, above, p. 62) tend to be associated with what have been termed 'line violations', in which closed systems are unnecessarily or carelessly broken into.

The bacteria typically responsible for cannula-related infections are

Table 4.4 The frequency of causative bacterial pathogens in septicaemia compared with the frequency in the more common kinds of HAI, from which it might have originated (data from NUH Singapore, 1986–9)

Pathogen	Percent infection caused by pathogens named					
	Sept	UTI	SWI	LRI	ICI	Skin
Gram-negative rods						
E. coli	14	23	8	2	2	3
Klebsiella spp.	21	21	11	11	7	6
P. aeruginosa	3	7	8	19	4	4
Acinetobacter spp.	4	4	4	8	10	2
Proteus spp.	1	7	3	3	1	5
Enterobacter spp.	3	2	3	2	0	1
Staph. aureus, ORSA	11	2	22	7	24	30
MARSA	11	3	18	25	26	29
Staph. epidermidis*	10	2	2	1	9	0
Streptococcus spp.	9	19	9	7	4	4
Candida spp.	6	4	3	8	8	10
Other pathogens	7	6	9	7	5	6

Staph. epidermidis is named here in the usual clinical sense, to include all coagulase-negative staphylococci except *Staph. saprophyticus*.
Key: Sept, septicaemia; UTI, urinary tract infection; SWI, surgical wound infection; LRI, lower respiratory infection; ICI, intravascular cannula-associated infection; Skin, skin infection.

shown in Table 4.4. Well over half of them are due to staphylococci. These normal inhabitants of the skin cause self- or cross-infections. Gram-negative bacteria may colonize the skin when it is wet and unhealthy, so infections with these bacteria may arise in the same way. Other potential sources are infections elsewhere in the patient. In this case, the bacteria responsible are likely to reach the cannula through the blood itself.

The longer an intravenous line is in place, the greater the chance that the inevitable superficial colonization of the puncture site will become an infection. Studies have shown that the number of infections begin to rise significantly after a cannula has been in place for 72 hours. This is why external lines should be changed at this point. If possible, the cannula and the site of cannulation are changed at the same time. This is often difficult, and in the case of central lines that must be maintained for a long time, perhaps impossible. Some central venous catheters for extended use are designed with cuffs that encourage the growth of tissue cells into them. The object is to form a living barrier to prevent the inevitable bacterial colonization at the puncture site from reaching the vein along the outside of the cannula.

Other methods that have been applied in an attempt to prevent cannula-related sepsis are the use of antiseptic ointments or occlusive dressings at the venipuncture site. Trials of antiseptics have given inconclusive results. This is not surprising, as these agents cannot sterilize the skin. Some occlusive dressings, particularly of an adhesive and perhaps transparent variety, have been shown to encourage an overgrowth of skin bacteria under them. They do this by providing the warm, moist environment bacteria love. The results of controlled trials of their use to cover intravascular penetration are not consistent. One reason for this may be that while both antiseptics and occlusive dressings might reduce sepsis due to cross-infection, neither is likely to have much effect on self-infection. The proportion of cannula-related infection attributable to intra- and extraluminal spread is likely to vary between hospitals. A trial done in a hospital where cross-infection contributes significantly to the total of cannula-related infections may show that antiseptics and occlusive dressings are effective. The opposite result is likely where procedures that minimize cross-infection are already in use.

Septicaemia

In this book, the term septicaemia is used to describe the presence of bacteria in the blood when this is accompanied by symptoms. Its symptomless counterpart is bacteraemia. Septicaemia is a common terminal event in overwhelming infections. Other than when bacteria are delivered from an external source by the intraluminal route, it must be inferred that they originate in an infection somewhere in the tissues of the body. In the context of HAI, septicaemia is most often secondary to urinary, surgical wound or lower-respiratory infections, or to extraluminal cannula-related sepsis. The state of the patient's immune system determines how severe a primary infection must be to cause septicaemia. In severe immunodeficiency, septicaemia may arise from a primary infection so inconspicuous that it cannot be located.

The bacteria identified as causing hospital acquired septicaemia in NUH are shown in Table 4.4. The bacteria found in some primary infections that might be the source of septicaemia are listed for comparison. There is an obvious connection between the distribution of bacterial pathogens in septicaemia and the four most frequent kinds of HAI. As septicaemia is nearly always secondary to infection elsewhere, control depends on preventing the primary cause.

Skin infections

For a significant part of the population *Staph. aureus* is a member of the normal flora of the skin (Table 2.3). It is also the principal cause of hospital acquired skin infections (Table 4.4). Table 2.4 shows that staphylococci cause more HAI in infants than is the case in children or adults. The figures are neonatal intensive care unit 48%, neonatal unit 56% (together 51%) compared with 22% for all other areas of the hospital. Figure 2.2 shows that 'other' infections are most common in the same two units. These are largely skin infections. The reason for this is that infants, born sterile, begin to develop their skin flora immediately they enter the world. They have to come to terms with *Staph. aureus*. Some achieve this without disease, but a significant number develop infections. Most of these are minor, but for two reasons it is important to keep them to a minimum. First, when staphylococcal colonization and infection rates rise in neonatal units, cases of serious staphylococcal sepsis begin to appear. Secondly, mothers who develop breast abscesses are nearly always infected with resistant hospital staphylococci acquired from their infants.

Gastrointestinal infections

The small number of gastrointestinal infections recorded in the NUH survey (Table 4.3) were due to rotaviruses, *Clostridium difficile*, and a few cases of antibiotic-associated diarrhoea in which heavy growths of *Aeromonas* spp. were interpreted as representing infections. There was one hospital-acquired infection due to a food-poisoning strain of salmonella. This was in an infant born to a mother who was just recovering from an infection with the same strain. This distribution of pathogens is not uncommon in gastrointestinal infections acquired in acute hospitals. However, in some parts of the world salmonellas are more important causes of HAI.

In the community, salmonella food poisoning is usually acquired from food that was contaminated at source. It has then been handled improperly so that a small innocuous dose of salmonellas is converted into a large infectious one, in the order of millions in a helping of contaminated foodstuff. This large dose is necessary if some are to survive the strong acid in the stomach and reach the intestine to start an infection there. Depending on the number of people who eat the contaminated food, the result will be a small or large outbreak of food poisoning. Secondary spread from person-to-person is uncommon, but may be seen within families, particularly where there are children.

Salmonellas may be introduced into a hospital in the same way as happens in the community, or a patient may be admitted who is already suffering from a salmonella infection. What happens next makes hospital outbreaks of salmonellosis different from those in the community. In long stay hospitals where mentally disturbed or retarded children or adults are cared for, it is possible to transmit the large infecting dose directly by the faecal-oral route. This cross-infection is the result of difficult hygienic conditions in these places, particularly if patients are suffering from diarrhoea. The situation is worse in psychogeriatric units because less gastric acid is produced in old age. This allows a smaller dose of salmonellas to start an infection, and so person-to-person transfer (cross-infection) is even easier.

In acute hospitals, direct person-to-person transfer of very large numbers of salmonellas is unlikely, but patients who are susceptible to smaller doses due to low gastric acidity are not uncommon. This is probably why infants can be infected by the small numbers of salmonellas carried on lightly contaminated hands. The same thing applies to anyone else who is producing less acid than normal because of debility or antacid treatment. When a significant number of patients who answer this description are found in one part of a hospital, salmonellas easily become entrenched there. A serious cross-infection problem can then develop as newly admitted patients keep the cycle of infection turning, and sooner or later members of staff are involved in the outbreak. It should be possible to control the situation by scrupulous attention to handwashing (staff **and** patients), but this may not be enforceable. It is often necessary to close the ward or wards involved to new admissions until the salmonella has burnt itself out and the remaining patients have been discharged.

The residual infections

These are made up of a small number of cases of HAI of many different kinds. With two exceptions, they are sufficiently like their community-acquired equivalents to require no further comment, except to note that they may be caused by hospital strains of bacteria.

The first exception involves medical devices made of plastic. *Staph. epidermidis* adheres strongly to the surface of plastic and multiplies there if the surrounding environment is nutritious. The association between plastic surfaces and *Staph. epidermidis* became obvious when shunts made of it were inserted to relieve hydrocephalus in infants with spina bifida. Shunts were frequently colonized. Antimicrobial treatment rarely worked and in the end they had to be removed. These colonizations and infections were nearly all self-infections, so control was difficult.

The second exception concerns infections of the eye. The inside of the eye is well protected from microbes, but once they gain entry it is poorly equipped to defend itself. If the resulting endophthalmitis is not energetically treated, the eye is usually destroyed. *Staph. aureus* and, particularly, *P. aeruginosa* are important pathogens in this situation. Postoperative endophthalmitis is very rare, but a perforated corneal ulcer can lead to it. *P. aeruginosa* and other pseudomonads may survive and even grow in solutions of the weak disinfectants used to preserve eye drops. It is possible to treat a patient with drops that contain a major pathogen for the eye without being aware of it, with potentially disastrous consequences. This is why eye drops must be sterilized carefully in small quantities for use on one occasion only, or for repeated use over a short period in the same patient. It is dangerous to use multi-dose containers of eye drops for several patients for periods of days or weeks. What has been said also applies to the solutions used by those who wear contact lenses.

Several diagnostic and therapeutic instruments used in ophthalmological practice touch the surface of the eye. Such apparatus, or at least that part of it that makes contact, must be sterilized or at least subjected to a high level of disinfection between uses. Failure to do this has in the past led to outbreaks of iatrogenic infection. The microbes involved have usually been viruses, adenoviruses in particular. On several occasions, tonometers have transferred infection from one patient to the eyes of others examined afterwards because of inadequate disinfection.

REFERENCES

Anon (1974) Microbiological hazards of intravenous infusions. *Lancet*, i, 543–4.

Cadwallader, H. L., Bradley, C. R. and Ayliffe, G. A. J. (1990) Bacterial contamination and frequency of changing ventilator circuitry. *J. Hosp. Infect.*, **15**, 65–72.

Colebrook, L. (1955) Infection acquired in hospital. *Lancet*, ii, 885–91.

Colebrook, L., Duncan J. M. and Ross W. P. D. (1948) The control of infection in burns. *Lancet*, i, 893–9.

Cruse, P. (1986) Surgical infection: incisional wounds, in *Hospital Infections*, 2nd edn, (eds J. V. Bennett and P. S. Brachman), Little Brown, Boston, pp. 423–36.

Krizek, T. J. and Robson, M. C. (1975) Biology of surgical infection. *Surgical Clin. N. America*, **55**, 1261–7.

Lidwell, O. M., Lowbury, E. J. L., Whyte, W. *et al.* (1982) Effect of ultraclean air in operating rooms on deep sepsis in the joint after total hip or knee replacement: a randomised study. *Br. Med. J.*, **285**, 10–4.

Meers, P. D. (1983a) Ventilation in operating rooms. *Br. Med. J.*, **286**, 244–5.

Meers, P. D. (1983b) Ventilation in operating rooms. *Br. Med. J.*, **286**, 1215.

Meers, P. D., Ayliffe, G. A. J., Emmerson, A. M. *et al.* (1981) National survey of infections in hospitals, 1980. *J. Hosp. Infect.*, **2** (Supplement), 23–8.

Miles, A. A. (1944) Epidemiology of wound infection. *Lancet*, **i**, 809–14.

Mishriki, S. F., Law, D. J. W. and Jeffrey, P. J. (1990) Factors affecting the incidence of postoperative wound infection. *J. Hosp. Infect.*, **16**, 223–30.

Mulhall, A. B., Chapman, R. G. and Crow, R. A. (1988) Bacteriuria during indwelling urethral catheterisation. *J. Hosp. Infect.*, **11**, 253–62.

National Research Council (1964) National Research Council uV study. *Ann. Surg.*, **160** (Supplement), 1–132.

Schweizer, R. T. (1976) Mask wiggling as a potential cause of wound contamination. *Lancet*, **ii**, 1129–30.

Stamm, W. E. (1986) Nosocomial urinary tract infections, in *Hospital Infections*, 2nd edn, (eds J. V. Bennett and P. S. Brachman), Little Brown, Boston, pp. 375–84.

Stickler, D. J. (1990) The role of antiseptics in the management of patients undergoing short-term indwelling bladder catheterisation. *J. Hosp. Infect.*, **16**, 89–108.

Warren, J. W. (1990) Nosocomial urinary tract infections, in *Priciples and Practice of Infectious Diseases*, 3rd edn, (eds G. L. Mandell, R. G. Douglas and J. E. Bennett), Churchill Livingstone, New York, pp. 2205–15.

Chapter 5

Practices in infection control

CARE OF THE HANDS

Everyone knows they should wash their hands after touching a patient, before going on to the next. Simple observation shows that this happens less often than it should. This impression is backed up by measurement. In a survey in an ICU, doctors were observed to wash their hands only 28 times out of each 100 occasions on which they should have done so. Comparable figures for nurses, radiographers and respiratory therapists were 43, 44, and 76 respectively. During the period of observation, hands were washed 494 times out of an ideal 1212 occasions. Because nurses touch patients more often than anyone else, they contributed 400 to the total of 718 failures to wash (Albert and Condie, 1981). However, nurses restrict their contacts to a small number of patients, and so the result of their failure is limited in its extent. Doctors tend to a larger number of more scattered patients, and so failure in their case is potentially more serious. In another study, a comparison was made between practices in an ICU before and after an upgrading that included an eightfold increase in the number of sinks for handwashing. The frequency of handwashing was a little higher in the new unit, rising to just 30% of the expected figure (Preston *et al.*, 1981)!

The purpose of handwashing is to remove dirt, and reduce the load of bacteria on the skin of the hands (Reybrouck, 1986). A wash with ordinary soap and water removes most of the transient bacterial flora. In hospitals, this includes important potential causes of handborne cross-infection (Chapter 2, p. 31). The resident flora of healthy hands is less likely to cause infection, except in immunocompromised patients. Resident bacteria are reduced in number by handwashing, particularly if a detergent containing an antiseptic is used, but they cannot be eliminated (Jarvis *et al.*, 1979). Even trivial injury to the skin alters the resident flora. Damage may be caused by failure to rinse the hands properly or, if they are not dried after washing, by the frequent use of strong detergents and antiseptics or by the vigorous use of a nail brush (Ojajarvi *et al.*, 1977). When the hands of hospital staff are damaged, the new and more numerous bacterial residents may include important causes of HAI. Washing even with an antiseptic does not remove resident bacteria old or new, and so staff in this condition are a serious threat to patients. Because the injuries are often inconspicuous, individuals may ignore or even be unaware of them, and unless they are tested bacteriologically they cannot know they are carrying an important pathogen (Meers and Leong, 1990).

Alcohol (spirit) is a powerful antiseptic that evaporates quickly. Applied to the skin it rapidly kills transient and a proportion of the resident bacteria, and then disappears. When it is desired to reduce the bacterial load on hands that are not soiled, washing can be replaced by the application of alcohol. The inclusion of a non-volatile antiseptic (chlorhexidine, for example) adds a residual effect to the immediate action of alcohol. If an emollient like glycerine and perhaps a perfume are added, the result is a de-germing lotion or handrub that when applied to the skin does not dry it too much (Kurtz and Boxall, 1976). A number of commercial products meet this specification. The wearing of gloves offers a third and most effective way of preventing the transfer of organisms to and from the hands.

A dilemma arises in areas like ICUs where the risk of HAI is high and handwashing ought to be more frequent. The use of disinfectant surgical scrubs is often encouraged in such places with the sensible intention of reducing the bacterial population of the hands. However, if this leads to damage to the skin, then the hands may be more dangerous than if ordinary soap had been used, or even if they had not been washed at all. A way out of the dilemma might be to provide several different handcare regimes in high-risk areas, to be used alternatively or sequentially at the discretion of members of staff or according to some protocol. The object would be to reduce the possibility of damage to the hands that can follow the repeated use of a single method on its own. Such techniques as washing with ordinary soap, with a surgical scrub, the use of a de-germing lotion, the wearing of gloves and the washing or antiseptic de-germing of gloved hands between procedures might be used in rotation, or as the task being performed dictates. In other clinical areas, handwashing with ordinary soap is all that is necessary, though the de-germing lotion has a place as a quick alternative for use during procedures that demand more than one handwash to complete them. De-germing lotions have a particular application where facilities for washing hands are inadequate.

Nail brushes should be used very little, and only to remove dirt that is ingrained or trapped under the nails. If employed at the same time as a strong detergent, damage to the skin is more likely. The traditional form of 'scrubbing up' in surgery probably does not improve on an energetic wash with an antiseptic detergent. A point worth remembering is that the water used for washing hands is rarely anything like sterile; indeed, it may contain surprisingly large numbers of bacteria. This is one of the reasons why a rub with alcohol (with or without added residual antiseptic) improves the hygiene of the hands after a surgical 'scrub'.

Hands are inseparable from health care. Hands are also recognized to be important causes of HAI. There is a general consensus that much of this HAI might be prevented by proper care, generally construed as more and better handwashing. Yet in practice it seems that hands are washed less than half as often as they should be. As this failure to wash was measured in an ICU where the importance of handwashing is likely to have been stressed, the situation may be worse in other parts of hospitals. The subject is ripe for a study of attitudes and motives. There is a need for more effective and less damaging handcare methods. Hot-air hand driers would lessen the damage done to hands by disposable towels made of the rougher kinds of paper. Their use would certainly reduce the volume of hospital waste, and perhaps reduce costs as well. Some newer models are less noisy than their predecessors, although they still take what may be thought an unacceptable time to dry the hands. This might deter some people from washing them in the first place. However, it should be noted that there are no **microbiological** contraindications to their use in clinical areas (Mathews and Newsom, 1987; Meers and Leong, 1989).

CATHETERS AND OTHER TUBES

Intravascular and urinary catheters, endotracheal and peritoneal dialysis tubes and the tubes used for drainage in surgery have several things in common. They all open ways into parts of the body from the outside, and so expose privileged surfaces and internal tissues (the forbidden zone) to microbes that are normally excluded (Figure 2.1). In this way, tubes allow microbes to reach, colonize and infect places that otherwise would be inaccessible to them. They give microbes a choice of routes by which to penetrate the body's normal defences, either round the outside of the tube (extraluminal) or by travelling through it (intraluminal). Infections that result from extraluminal spread are almost entirely endogenous (or autogenous) self-infections. Infections following intraluminal spread are usually exogenous, the microbes concerned arriving as a result of cross-infection or environmental infection (Figure 2.4).

Depending on circumstances, the extraluminal (endogenous or autogenous) route of infection may be more or less common than the intraluminal (exogenous) route. There are a number of important variables. These are, first, if the tube is filled with liquid or air and the direction of flow, secondly, the weight of colonization of the body surface at the point of entry or exit of the tube and, thirdly, the level of care exercised in the insertion and management of the system. Colonization and infection of that part of the forbidden zone entered by the tube becomes increasingly common as time passes. To slow this down or prevent it requires an assessment to be made to determine which route of infection is more important. This is a job for the ICT, which should also recommend procedures to reduce the risk. Control measures designed to delay the appearance of infection vary according to the route by which the contaminating microbes gain entry. Most tubes are left in place for a very few days. In these cases, management that delays the entry of bacteria by the most important route will be cost-effective if the tube has been removed by the time infection would otherwise have been a serious threat. It is also useful for staff to understand how infections develop so that frustration is less likely to dampen enthusiasm for attempts at control.

Control of the extraluminal routes have been discussed in the various sections of Chapter 4. The methods can be summarized as choice of tube, care at insertion, the use of antiseptics, and maintenance. The materials used in the construction of the tube and its size may be important. Insertion should be made with the least possible trauma, to limit damage to the body's innate defences. Where possible, the body surface through which the tube is to be introduced should be carefully cleaned and disinfected. This is to reduce the number of bacteria carried on the outside of the tube when it is inserted into the forbidden zone. For skin disinfection, quick-acting alcoholic solutions are preferred. On mucous membranes, less-effective and more slowly acting aqueous solutions have to be used. Compared to the nearly instantaneous effect of alcohol, these take some minutes to produce the desired result. Whatever procedure is planned it should not start until the necessary time has passed.

It is not clear if regular toilet of the skin round insertion sites is of use, or if antiseptic ointments should be applied to them. Fiddling with the entry point increases the risk of infection with urinary catheters, and so meatal toilet as a special procedure is not encouraged. Washing to a good standard of personal hygiene is sufficient. By extension these considerations may apply to tubes of other kinds. Although the application of antiseptic ointments is controversial (Chapter 4, p. 84), topical ointments containing antimicrobial drugs should never be used as they encourage the appearance of resistant strains of bacteria.

Maintenance may be summarized as keeping closed systems closed as much as possible, the use of careful, clean techniques when it is necessary to break into closed systems, and adherence to the best advice on the frequency of changing tubes and their associated external apparatus. The latter is doubly important as significant sums of money can be saved by not changing complex and expensive apparatus as often as has sometimes been advocated in the past.

Intraluminal spread varies in importance. The application of inadequate procedures for the care of urinary catheters is accompanied by unacceptable rates of colonization and infection. This is usually due to contamination by the intraluminal route. It is silly to buy modern apparatus for the collection of urine by the closed method, and use it so that the system is effectively open. Intraluminal spread is usually less of a problem with other tubes that contain liquids, because more attention is paid to them. From the point of view of preventing infection, an intravenous drip and a urine collecting system deserve the same level of care.

Tubes of the kinds under consideration have a potential for doing good and harm. To some extent, harm (in this context, the development of infection) is unavoidable and has to be accepted as the price of doing good. Sensible, well thought-out procedures that are understood and followed by everyone keep harm to a minimum. The incidence of infection associated with the use of tubes increases with time. The length of time between insertion of a tube and the development of an infection can be increased if control measures are applied. If a patient's tube is no longer needed and it is taken out before an infection has time to appear, that patient is spared HAI. Once a tube has been inserted, it should be reviewed regularly to see if it can be removed. It cannot be stressed too much that all these tubes are potential killers. They should not be used for convenience.

ISOLATION

Background

The application of isolation to the control of infection has its roots in antiquity. The human race has always over-reacted to dangers it does not comprehend. Lepers and sufferers from bubonic plague, for instance, were isolated from the community. Although this may have done something for general peace of mind, it did nothing to prevent the spread of either disease. The segregation of people to stop the spread of contagion and the enforcement of quarantine evolved as described in Chapters 1 (p. 3) and 3 (p. 48). Although the original work of Semmelweis and Lister had dealt with specific and classical forms of HAI, emphasis was soon diverted towards the control of such epidemic forms of CAI as cholera and diphtheria. Interest in the control of HAI did not resurface until the 1940s. At the time, barrier nursing was one of the methods thought appropriate to prevent the spread of CAI when a case of it was admitted to hospital. Later, barrier nursing (renamed isolation) was adapted to the control of HAI as well. Many senior nurses had worked in fever hospitals, and so the various techniques of barrier nursing were transferred as they stood.

By the 1960s, the need for standardization was apparent, and in 1970 the CDC published a handbook on isolation techniques, with a revision in 1975. These described various categories of isolation appropriate to the supposed route of transmission of each infection. During the 1970s, attention was increasingly focussed on HAI, and more was learnt about its epidemiology. It became apparent that the requirements for isolation were too rigorous, and in 1983 new recommendations were issued (Garner and Simmons, 1983, 1986). HAI was now dealt with more fully, but the recommendations still concentrated on such CAIs as tuberculosis, hepatitis B and varicella-zoster. In many places, these had by now become minor components of HAI, though this was not true everywhere.

In 1987, a new approach to the control of the spread of HAI was proposed. This was originally called body substance isolation, though it soon developed into universal precautions (Lynch *et al.*, 1987; Centers for Disease Control, 1988). The major stimulus was anxiety about the presence of undiagnosed cases of hepatitis B and HIV infection in hospitals. It emphasized the application of relatively simple barrier precautions (wearing gloves, for instance) for **every** patient when contact is made with potentially infected (and so all) body secretions. The need for true isolation in a single room was reduced to a short list of what for most hospitals were uncommon conditions. This approach has not been accepted universally and some hospitals have developed a two-tier system. This combines universal precautions with a variable residue of earlier practices.

It is difficult for hospitals to adopt a complete, ready-made package of isolation procedures. Each needs to evolve its own set, or at least modify an existing one, according to circumstances. The development of an isolation policy is an important task for the ICT and the ICC.

Basics

It is sometimes thought necessary to care for patients under conditions of physical isolation. This may be complete, or apply only to one or more kinds of interpersonal contact. A patient with an infection may be isolated from other patients and staff, who otherwise might catch it (**source isolation**, equivalent to the old barrier nursing). Alternatively, a specially susceptible patient may be isolated to protect him or her from an infection carried by others (**protective isolation**, originally called reverse barrier nursing).

To be successful, source isolation depends on the person (or persons) isolated being the only source of the unwanted pathogenic microbe in the hospital. This may be true with cases of Lassa fever or diphtheria, for example. It is clearly not true for most cases of HAI that are caused by microbes that are more or less widely distributed in the hospital or the community, either in carriers or in cases of clinical or sub-clinical infections. There is very little to be gained by isolating a patient with a MARSA infection, for instance, unless it is certain that all the others who carry the same organism (patients **and** staff) are isolated or excluded simultaneously. Isolation may be of limited value if the person isolated is an unusually prolific source of the pathogen concerned. In general, however, unless a complete barrier is erected between all who carry the microbe to be excluded and those who do not, the exercise tends to be an expensive ritual. A major weakness of isolation (for patients) or exclusion (for staff) is that in most cases neither can begin until a microbiological examination has shown the need for it. During the 24–48 hours delay this imposes, the pathogen to be isolated or excluded may already have spread to others.

If a significant number of patients are colonized or infected with a pathogen that ought to be isolated, a system of cohort nursing can be instituted. All the patients affected are moved to a discrete clinical area where they are cared for by nurses who are restricted to these patients. In this way, nurses who are themselves carriers of the unwanted pathogen may continue to be employed rather than being excluded from the hospital. Of course, this can only work if the cohort includes **all** who are infected with the pathogen, plus those who are carrying it. This implies a large-scale microbiological investigation so that everyone is allocated to the correct category.

The features of complete isolation include the use of a single room with an air-lock ante-room containing a handbasin for staff use, provided with a toilet bay containing another handbasin, water closet and shower for the patient. The air supply may be at slightly reduced pressure for source isolation with discharge into the open away from people or air inlets. For protective isolation, the air pressure in the room may be kept a little above atmospheric. Staff should, of course, wash their hands on entering and leaving, and depending on local rules may be required to don gowns, aprons, masks or gloves in the ante-room, and remove them when they leave. As well as regulating these factors, rules may also be made about who and what can enter or leave the room, and in the case of source isolation, how anything leaving is wrapped, and how it is treated at its destination.

The most complete form of isolation is provided in specialist infectious disease units. Here even the staff caring for the patient may be isolated from the rest of the world, as used to happen with smallpox. In extreme cases, a plastic isolator may be used that completely encloses the patient and his or her bed. The patient is cared for through armholes fitted with long-sleeved gloves. Food, drugs and other items are passed in and out through an airlock. Fresh air is pumped into the isolation capsule, filtered on its way out in the case of source isolation, or on its way in for the protective form.

In the past, protective isolation has been used mainly for patients who are immunosuppressed for transplantation. As immuno-suppression for this purpose has become more sophisticated, and with growing experience, several major centres have reduced the level of isolation they require for these patients. Many of the extreme requirements, such as rooms ventilated with ultra-clean (laminar flow) air, the provision of sterilized food, prohibition of physical contact with others, and the extensive use of prophylactic antimicrobials or anti-septics, have been abandoned. Even single-room isolation is not always considered necessary, provided handwashing is rigorously enforced. Opinions vary about this. Individual decisions may turn on such factors as where in the hospital the isolation area is located. If it is in a surgical ICU with a high incidence of HAI more protection may be called for. One of the reasons for the general relaxation of precautions is the observation that infections in many of these patients are self-infections.

Source isolation developed in two different ways. In the 1983 CDC category-specific variety, seven different types of isolation are defined. For each a separate list of procedures is laid down. Many hospitals have developed equivalent systems, but with only three or four categories. The CDC system is outlined in Table 5.1. As the precautions in each category have been designed to meet worst-case conditions, for the average situation they are too demanding. The need for the full list of recommendations is not everywhere accepted, and the diseases for which isolation is suggested include a number that are not thought to require special precautions in much of the world. Many

Table 5.1 An outline of the precautions recommended by CDC for category-specific isolation

Isolation category	Types of infection
A. Strict isolation:	Disseminated varicella-zoster, pneumonic plague: for Lassa fever etc., change 2* in Table below to 3.
B. Contact isolation:	Paediatric patients with acute respiratory infections; neonates with gonococcal conjunctivitis, herpes simplex or staphylococcal skin infection; any patient with cutaneous diphtheria, disseminated herpes, infection or colonization by epidemiologically significant multiple resistant bacteria, staphylococcal pneumonia or major skin infections or infestations, rubella, vaccinia.
C. Respiratory isolation:	Measles, erythema infectiosum, respiratory infection including meningitis due to *Haemophilus influenzae* invasive meningococcal disease, mumps, pertussis.
D. Tuberculosis isolation:	Actual or suspected open (infectious) tuberculosis
E. Enteric precautions:	Infectious gastrointestinal disease, including hepatitis A.
F. Drainage-secretion precautions:	Any disease producing an infective purulent discharge, unless already in a more demanding category
G. Blood–body fluid:	HIV infection, arthropod-borne viral fevers, hepatitis B, non-A non-B, leptospirosis, malaria, etc.

Requirements	Isolation categories						
	A	B	C	D	E	F	G
Separate room	2*	2	2	3	1	0	1
Gowns	2	1	0	1	1	1	1
Gloves	2	1	0	0	1	1	1
Masks	2	1	1	4	0	0	0
Handwashing	2	1	1	1	1	1	1
Waste and equipment	6	6	6	5	6	6	6

0 = Not necessary
1 = Optional, or only in connection with direct patient contact
2 = Necessary
3 = Room with special ventilation
4 = Masks worn if patient coughing
5 = Waste and other fomites treated as mildly infective
6 = As for 5, but special decontamination for reusable items

hospitals would find it difficult to apply the full CDC recommendations for lack of sufficient isolation accommodation.

In disease-specific source isolation, the precautions are individual to each infection, according to its 'infectiousness' and the route by which it spreads. This makes it more flexible and less wasteful than category-specific isolation, but the choice of the appropriate set of precautions requires a degree of specialist knowledge and skill that often prevents categorization by ward staff. The CDC recommendations list over 160 different diseases or conditions, each with its own precautions (Garner and Simmons, 1986). Members of the ICT usually need to be involved with each decision. This may not be easy at night or at weekends.

It is a fact that although many regard isolation as central to the control of infection, good evidence of its efficacy is lacking. This is a pity, because isolation is expensive. It is likely to damage patients' mental health, and may damage their physical health as well if isolation deprives them of any special monitoring or treatment they need. The general tendency over recent years has been to relax requirements for isolation. It is probable that this trend will continue. Because airborne and other environmental sources are of small importance as causes of infection, it is very uncertain that single-room isolation is really necessary other than in extreme situations (Lassa fever, for example). It may be that the contribution of isolation is to provide a physical barrier that reminds staff to apply the precautions that they ought to be using for all patient contact.

The lack of hard logic makes drawing up an isolation policy one of the more difficult tasks that faces infection control organizations in hospitals. Not least among the problems is the need to identify which members of staff are to initiate isolation and define its extent in each case. Attempts to import ready-made solutions are likely to fall foul of local conditions, and will almost certainly lead to over-isolation, unnecessary expense and, perhaps, failure if inadequate resources are overextended. There is no doubt that subconscious fear of infection keeps alive the mystery and ritual that surrounds much of the practice of isolation. Education and the application of scientifically based common sense are the answers to this.

DRESSING SURGICAL WOUNDS

This section should be read in conjunction with Chapters 4 (p. 64) and 6 (p. 131). It is necessary to stress again the important distinction to be made between wounds that are 'closed' because their skin edges have been brought together accurately and intimately (typically at the end of an operation), and those which are 'open'. Open wounds range from surgical incisions that were originally closed, but where the suture line has broken down or where primary closure was undesirable or impossible, to pressure sores, ulcers of different kinds, and burns (Chapter 6, p. 140). These two types of wound differ fundamentally in their potential for bacterial colonization and infection and the rates at which they heal, and how this happens. These differences are so great that the nursing attention applied to each might also be different. In Chapters 1 (p. 7) and 4 (p. 65) the introduction of the 'no-touch' dressing technique was related to infections in war wounds. These were open wounds. The question then is, is it necessary to employ a technique that was invented for the dressing of open wounds to the usually more numerous closed variety? It seems that large sums of money might be saved if simplified methods were used for dressing the latter. This has been achieved in some hospitals (Chapter 4, p. 69).

Most operative wounds are closed completely at the end of surgery, with or without a vacuum drain. If such a wound breaks down later, the cause was nearly always present within it at the time the patient left the operating room. A surgical problem is the usual underlying cause (Chapter 4, p. 69). If an infection develops in a wound in which the soil (tissue) has been fertilized (made more susceptible) in this way, a relatively small dose of bacterial seed planted at the same time may be enough to start an infection. Probably less often the seed travels through the blood to settle in the fertilized soil some time later. The source of the bacteria in these haematogenous infections is likely to have been a septic condition elsewhere in the body – a urinary tract infection, for example.

After a few hours, wounds that have been completely closed are effectively sealed to the entry of bacteria from the outside (see Chapter 4, p. 69, for more details). Because subcutaneous tissues are not exposed in these wounds, there is none of the desiccation that is thought to delay healing. In these circumstances, what happens in the ward postoperatively has little bearing on whether closed surgical wounds become infected or the rate at which they heal. They do not need to be dressed using an elaborate and expensive so-called aseptic (sterile) technique. A simple clean procedure is all that is required. The dressing applied in the operating room may be kept in place for longer, or the changing procedure simplified, or both.

Wounds in which subcutaneous tissues are exposed without a covering of skin are completely different. Bacterial colonization or infection is inevitable and healing, perhaps already slowed down by a poor blood supply, may be compromised further by desiccation. The deleterious effect of the latter has attracted attention recently, and the correction of this by the use of appropriate dressings together with other new developments may have improved the outlook for the healing of these wounds. This is of interest microbiologically, because a wound dressed so that it is kept moist provides an environment in which bacteria will grow more freely. Some years ago open wounds, particularly burns, were treated by exposure expressly to prevent this, by keeping them as dry as possible.

In most cases, the first bacteria to colonize an open wound are derived from the patient's own microbial flora. This may contribute a hospital strain of bacteria if the patient's normal flora has been altered because he or she has already spent some time in hospital. The patient may be nursed in an area where there are a number of others with similar wounds. In such cases, it has proved difficult or impossible to prevent the 'personal' bacteria of the initial colonization from being replaced by multi-resistant hospital strains of bacteria that typically infest such clinical areas. The tendency for all the open wounds in the same clinical area to be colonized or infected by the same bacteria is best seen in burns units. What determines the point at which a colonization becomes an infection in an open wound is unknown. Stratagems for diagnosing and treating these infections are complex, and best determined in the context of local conditions.

Changing the dressings on open wounds requires the use of a sterile, no-touch technique, because the exudate probably contains large numbers of bacteria, which may be of undesirable, multi-resistant hospital strains. When wounds of both types are present in the same clinical area, it makes microbiological sense if those that are classified as open are dressed after any closed ones have been dealt with. This separation is a good idea because the various techniques used to prevent the transfer of bacteria between patients (no-touch, gloves and handwashing) are less than perfect. Even if handwashing fails, is incomplete or even forgotten, the error is more likely to be forgiven if the hands have not yet been contaminated from an infected wound. The purpose is to avoid spreading hospital strains of bacteria to patients or staff who are still free of them.

The same logic applies to the dressing of open wounds. If possible they should be dressed in the order: wounds with open (corrugated or Yeates) drains not known to be infected or colonized; wounds colonized or infected with bacteria that are not hospital strains; wounds that are already colonized or infected with a hospital strain of bacteria. Of course, if there are enough nurses and ward routine allows, a different nurse can attend to each class of wound, or one can attend to the open variety while another is dealing with closed wounds.

If it is desired to avoid the waste inherent in approaching all wounds as if they required to be dealt with by a classical no-touch technique, a decision has to be made in each case. There is no problem with wounds known to be open. Difficulty arises because the condition of a wound closed primarily, with or without vacuum drainage, usually cannot be assessed until the dressing is removed. If the dressing is wet, then the wound is assumed to be infected, and a sterile procedure appropriate to an open wound is employed. If the dressing is dry, it can be lifted wearing a clean plastic bag drawn on to the dominant hand in preference to a more expensive glove. The old dressing is removed and the bag is turned inside out over it for discard. Whatever attention is thought necessary is performed as a simple clean (not sterile) procedure, and another dressing applied if required. If the wound is found to be infected, it is re-covered temporarily and the patient, now consigned to the group with open wounds, is dealt with a little later using a sterile procedure.

It is appropriate to use either gloves or forceps in a sterile procedure. If disposable gloves are chosen they need not have been sterilized, and there is no reason to buy an expensive variety. Cheap plastic gloves from a responsible supplier that are intended for clinical use are virtually free of microbes when taken from their packs, provided these have been designed sensibly. They should emerge through a small opening in their box, and be packed within it so that each protects the one below. Nurses changing dressings should wear plastic aprons to protect their clothing from splashes. These need not be changed between patients when dealing with closed wounds, but they should be changed between dressing open ones. If this is inappropriate due to cost or the fear of producing too much plastic waste, a fresh clean (not necessarily sterile) fabric gown may be used for each patient, worn over a plastic apron that is not changed. However, it is important to recognize that gowns made of ordinary fabrics cannot prevent bacteria contained in splashes or carried on skin squames from passing through them (Chapter 6, p. 132). Without a plastic apron underneath, they offer no useful protection, either to the wearer or the wound. The plastic apron is likely to be contaminated if the gown over it gets wet, and so this alternative is less attractive than a plastic apron that is changed between patients with open wounds. Of course, nurses should wash their hands between each procedure. Masks are unnecessary.

A good deal of folklore attaches to the possibility of bacteria being carried from patient to patient on nurses' clothing. Clean clothing that has been properly laundered (Chapter 7, p. 152) is virtually sterile. If it remains dry, any of the small number of bacteria that adhere to it during wear do not survive well. In the absence of major soiling with faeces, heavily infected urine or frank pus, clothing will always have many fewer bacteria on it than are present on the skin of the wearer under it. The transfer of bacteria from a nurse's clothing to a wound requires that direct physical contact is made between the two. Bacteria cannot jump, nor are they easily detached from surfaces once they have arrived there, and so for practical purposes spread from clothing through the air is not a problem.

Dressings fulfil a fivefold purpose. First, they should protect a wound from infection from the outside for the few hours to a number of days (depending on the type) during which this remains a possibility. Secondly, with open wounds they should produce the physical conditions under them required to promote rapid healing. Thirdly, they should soak up any discharge from the wound. Fourthly, they act to prevent stitches or clips catching on clothing etc. Fifthly, they keep prying fingers at bay.

The importance or otherwise of dressings on closed surgical wounds is highlighted by a report of a trial in which surgical wounds of this type were left undressed, without harm to patients (Howells and Young, 1966). After the first few hours, it may be that the presence of a dressing on a closed wound fulfils a psychological rather than any real need.

WEARING MASKS

In the medical context, face masks are worn to protect patients from microbes expelled from the respiratory tract of members of staff, or to protect wearers from a source of airborne microbes. In both cases, the purpose is to prevent infection. There is no evidence that wearing them achieves this objective, but there is some evidence that infection does not increase if they are **not** worn. This measure for the control of infection, apparently first introduced into surgery intuitively at the end of the nineteenth century, has become an entrenched ritual.

It has been shown that counts of aerial bacteria in ORs are the same no matter if masks are worn or not (Ritter et al., 1974). A surgical team that operated for a period of six months without masks (432 surgical wounds) noted a slight reduction in the rate of SWI compared with the same period in each of the previous four years when masks were worn (Orr, 1981). It has been found that infection rates are unchanged whether or not masks are worn when dressing wounds (Gillespie et al., 1959), and that they are not important in isolation nursing (Ayliffe et al., 1979) or in the delivery room (Turner et al., 1984). In the face of this sort of evidence, the efficiency of masks as bacterial filters is of no relevance, although manufacturers use this as a selling point. If they are to be worn at all, there seems to be no reason to spend a lot of money on them.

The rationale for this is the fact that very few bacteria are shed from the mouth and nose when breathing and talking normally, and even among these few, pathogens are rare (Duguid, 1946). Coughing and particularly sneezing produce larger numbers, but these are as likely to emerge round the edges of masks as to be filtered out by them. Because a proportion of inspired air also passes round the edges of masks, they provide less protection to the wearer than might be supposed. It has already been noted that the inevitable rubbing of masks on the face releases potentially infected skin squames (Chapter 4, p. 74). It is easy to imagine where the larger of these get to in the case of a surgeon looking vertically down into a wound.

Rationalization to the point that masks are abandoned altogether is unlikely to be achieved, not least because many of those who are accustomed to wearing them enjoy doing so. However, it should be possible to restrict their use quite drastically, and so save a great deal of money. This would also reduce the need to point out that the improper use of masks is itself a hazard. It would be an advance if staff were no longer seen carrying masks in their pockets, or wearing them round their necks, or adjusting them with hands that are used immediately afterwards to touch a patient.

DISABLING OR KILLING MICROBES

Without microbes, there would be no infections, but as life as we know it on earth would be impossible without them, they must not be killed indiscriminately. Any necessary killing should be selective, designed to inactivate or destroy the few kinds of microbes that might harm us. This is difficult because microbes share with us and with animals and plants most of the processes that together constitute 'life'. The result is that the most effective ways of killing microbes are also lethal to other living things. Each of us is home to many millions of microbes, and so we have to come to terms with them. Attempts to harm any of them must be carefully designed and applied to avoid (so far as possible) damage to ourselves, remembering that microbes can adapt to new surroundings more cleverly and much more quickly than we can. Microbes are likely to remain on earth long after man has disappeared from it.

The word 'disabling' is included in the title of this section for two reasons. First, as viruses are not truly alive they cannot be killed, but they may be disabled or inactivated so they can no longer multiply to cause infections. Secondly, some useful antimicrobial drugs can do no more than stop bacteria multiplying. If an infection is treated with one of these, the body depends on its normal defences to kill and clear away the residue. A difficulty that arises in discussing the destruction of microbes is that, in the human context, the words 'alive' or 'dead' are nearly always perceived to relate to individuals one at a time. Microbes must be thought of in whole populations, numbered in millions. Even if 99% of a million germs are killed, 10 000 are left alive. After an hour in the right circumstances, this residue can again number a million.

As with any form of life gathered together in large numbers, populations of microbes do not respond immediately or consistently to toxic or lethal agents. There are very large differences in the sensitivity of different kinds of microbe to the same agent, and even within a

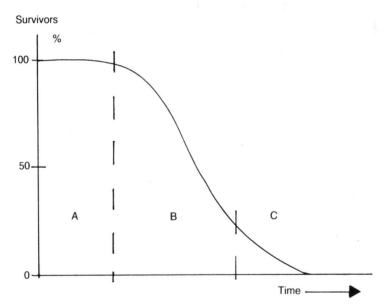

Figure 5.1 The result of applying a disabling or killing agent to a population of microbes, at the beginning of period 'A'. During the remainder of this period, the agent is reaching its target and beginning to have an effect. During period 'B' killing or disabling is achieved and then progresses at a steady rate, and in period 'C' more resistant or inaccessible microbes are dealt with. Period 'A + B + C' may measure minutes, hours or last for ever, depending on the power of the agent and the resistance of the microbe.

population of a single type of microbe, significant variations in sensitivity are found. The power of toxic or lethal agents also varies, for two reasons. Some are intrinsically more active than others, and they may be applied differently (more or less hot, more or less concentrated or diluted, for longer or shorter periods, etc.). Because of this, the outcome of their use can only be predicted in a general way. With very powerful agents, the unpredictability is less than with weaker ones and, as they get weaker, other factors like the presence of dirt become progressively more important in determining if the process succeeds or fails in its purpose.

Figure 5.1 displays the result of applying a killing agent to a population of microbes. This so-called 'killing curve' is divided into three parts. First, the killing agent must penetrate to reach the target where it is to act to kill or disable each microbe, and then begin to have an effect. This takes time, represented by part 'A' of the curve. With powerful agents, this may be very short – measured in seconds. With weaker agents, it may measure minutes or hours or, of course, if the organism is resistant to the agent, it lasts for ever. Part 'B' of the curve depicts the steady killing (or disablement) of sensitive microbes. The slope of this part of the curve is more or less steep depending on the rate of killing, which varies with the power of the agent and the resistance of the microbe. In part 'C' of the curve, slightly more resistant microbes take longer to die. With more resistant microbes and weaker agents, the curve may fail to reach the baseline, implying that some microbes survive the process. In different circumstances, the time A + B + C can vary from seconds to infinity.

The principal factors that determine the outcome when a toxic or lethal agent is applied to a population of microbes are the power of the killing agent and the resistance of the microbe. As an example of the variability of these factors, the sensitivity of different microbes to heat is illustrated in Table 5.2. A similar table drawn up for exposure to

Table 5.2 An indication of the sensitivity of different microbes to heat

Killing (disabling) by moist heat		
Easy 60–80°C	*Intermediate 80–100°C*	*Difficult – longer at 100°C or >100°C*
Most vegetative bacteria, many viruses	Some vegetative bacteria and spores, some viruses and fungi	Some spores, viroids, prions

toxic chemicals would show the length of exposure and/or its concentration as the variable in the place of temperature. There would be significant changes in the contents of the boxes representing the three categories of killing. For instance, the tubercle bacillus, which falls in the 'easy' category for heat, would move to the 'difficult' one for many of the stronger chemical disinfectants, and to a new fourth category ('impossible') for weaker ones.

It is customary to divide the agencies or agents used to kill or disable microbes into those that 'sterilize' and those that 'disinfect'. Sterilization is often defined as a process designed to destroy all living things. Microbiological sterility is the total absence of microbes able to reproduce themselves. A sterilized product is, therefore, no longer infectious, though it may still be toxic due to the presence of dead microbes or parts of them.

In practice, the definition breaks down because the requirement for absolute and total destruction is unattainable (Kelsey, 1972). It is possible to design tests so severe that if they were used all normal sterilizing methods would fail. To overcome this largely theoretical difficulty, it has generally been accepted that sterilization is achieved by a process that reliably and reproducibly kills something approaching one million resistant bacterial spores. For steam sterilizers, spores of the heat-resistant *Bacillus stearothermophilus* are used. The unsatisfactory nature of this definition is underlined by the fact that 'sterilization' in an autoclave even to this quite severe standard does not destroy the infectivity of material containing the agents of the spongiform encephalopathies, of which Creutzfeldt–Jakob disease is a human variety and 'mad-cow disease' (bovine spongiform encephalopathy) another example. These and similar agents called viroids or prions may require to be autoclaved for six times the normal period to inactivate them.

Processes that kill or inactivate useful numbers of microbes, but cannot reliably produce complete sterilization, are called **disinfecting methods**. Diagnostic or therapeutic instruments intended for invasive use should ideally be sterile. Because some of them are made of materials, or mixtures of materials, that would be damaged or destroyed by sterilization, they are disinfected instead. To be effective, a disinfecting agent must reduce the number of microbes present on or in an object intended for clinical use, or that may be found on a body surface or in tissue, to a level that is harmless in the context concerned, and for the purpose intended. What is 'harmless' is difficult to define, not least because a small number of residual microbes that may be harmless to a healthy adult may injure an immunocompromised patient being treated in hospital. Careful attention to the 'purpose intended' is there-

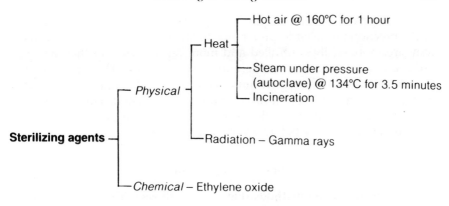

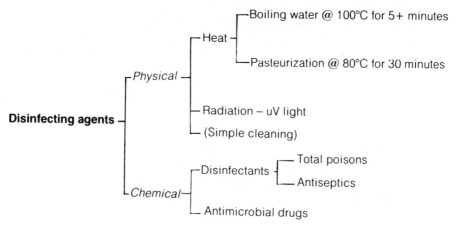

Figure 5.2 Flow chart summarizing sterilizing and disinfecting methods commonly used in medical practice.

fore important. Chemical disinfecting agents are called **disinfectants**. If a disinfectant is sufficiently non-toxic to be used on skin, mucous membranes or exposed tissue, it is called an **antiseptic**.

Figure 5.2 summarizes the sterilizing and disinfecting methods commonly used in hospitals, or by the suppliers of materials used in medical practice.

In all disinfection and sterilization practice, it is important to ensure that objects to be treated are as clean as possible before they are exposed to the process. Cleaning alone usually removes many of the microbes initially present on or in them, and so reduces the chances of failure when they are sterilized, or allows disinfection to be more complete. As disinfecting methods get weaker, prior cleaning becomes more important. Whenever possible, physical methods of sterilization or disinfection are used in preference to chemical ones. This is because they are more easily controlled and more reproducible in their action. They are also usually cheaper and may be safer. They may allow treatment to be completed within a wrapping, and so the process ends with a dry sterile object that can be stored until needed. This is not true of chemical methods in which toxic liquids are employed, as these must be washed away before an object can be used.

Sterilizing methods

Among the sterilizing methods (Figure 5.2), those with a physical basis are generally more powerful, and so have a wider margin of safety and are more convenient to use than the chemical ones. Chemical methods are used only when items to be sterilized are made of materials or mixtures of materials that will not withstand, or for some reason cannot be exposed to, physical methods. The requirement for sterility as defined is imposed by the need to destroy the most resistant microbial forms. Until recently, these were thought to be bacterial spores, particularly those of *Clostridium tetani*, the cause of tetanus. For most other microbes, sterilization represents massive overkill, and so provides a wide safety margin. The growing interest in viroids and prions in human, animal and plant pathology has yet to be reflected in routine sterilizing or disinfecting practice. There will be far-reaching changes if it becomes necessary to take account of these unusual infectious agents.

Hot-air ovens
Although hot-air (or more sophisticated infra-red) ovens are comparatively cheap and simple to use, they have almost disappeared from hospitals. This is because the number of reusable items in clinical practice that require to be sterilized and that can withstand heating to 160°C or more without damage is now very small. Another difficulty is that wrappings made even of kraft paper become brittle and fabrics are damaged at these temperatures. To prevent recontamination before use, items sterilized in hot-air ovens are often packed in custom-made containers usually made of metal.

A hot-air oven resembles a domestic oven fitted with a fan to ensure the even distribution of heat to all parts of the chamber. An accurate thermometer or, better, a recording thermometer regularly checked for its precision is required as necessary instrumentation. In use, the oven must not be packed tightly, so that the hot air can penetrate to heat the load as evenly and quickly as possible. Timing of the sterilizing cycle starts when the temperature has reached the desired level: 160°C for one hour is usual for small items that heat up quickly. The use of biological controls (spores) is not necessary as a routine, as the physical parameters (temperature and time) are well established. When a new oven is used for the first time, or an unusually large or complex item has to be sterilized by hot air, spore strips containing *B. subtilis* may be included initially to validate the process or, in the second case, to determine if times in excess of an hour are required to allow for full penetration by heat. The spores are placed within the packets to be sterilized, or in the internal parts of more complex objects. Alternatively, the temperatures may be measured with thermocouples, or use made of the commercially available indicators that incorporate heat-sensitive materials that change their colour or form to show that a certain temperature has been achieved. The latter need to be used with care, as improper storage, for instance, may change their sensitivity.

Steam under pressure: the steam sterilizer or autoclave
Autoclaves are the mainstay of sterilizing practice in nearly all hospitals. Most reusable items can be sterilized in them, with notable exceptions such as apparatus containing heat-sensitive optical or electronic components (endoscopes or pacemakers), or things made of the kinds of plastic that soften at lower temperatures. An autoclave is significantly more expensive and potentially more dangerous than a hot-air oven. A modern fully automatic autoclave is a very complicated piece of machinery that requires regular maintenance by an expert engineer. Despite this, the physical principles that govern the operation of autoclaves are not complex, and to avoid elementary mistakes the basis of these should be understood by those who superintend their use.

A hot-air oven takes an hour to produce sterility at 160°C, while an autoclave can do the same in just 3.5 minutes at a lower temperature (134°C). The following facts explain the difference.

1. Saturated steam condenses on anything cooler than itself, instantly releasing its latent heat of vaporization and so rapidly raising the temperature of the surface concerned. (Compare putting your hand into a domestic oven at say 200°C with the effect on your skin of steam from the spout of a kettle at half the temperature.)
2. As steam condenses to water, it contracts to a tiny fraction of its former volume. The partial vacuum created draws in more steam and the process is repeated until the object being sterilized has reached the temperature of the steam and condensation ceases.
3. The temperature of steam rises as the pressure is increased. At

atmospheric pressure, steam is at 100°C, at twice and three times this pressure, the temperatures are 121°C and 134°C respectively.

It follows from (1) and (2) that steam can only sterilize surfaces it can reach. Objects enclosed in wrappings or boxes through which steam cannot penetrate are, in effect, being exposed as if they were in a hot-air oven. Because of the lower temperature and the shorter time used in autoclaves, sterilization will not be achieved. Steam operates much more effectively if substantially all the air is removed from the chamber of an autoclave before sterilization commences. Modern autoclaves are equipped to produce an efficient vacuum in the chamber before admitting the sterilizing steam. This is particularly important for autoclaves intended for sterilizing wrapped objects, the so-called 'porous load' sterilizers. At the end of a sterilizing cycle, there is a vacuum inside the chamber which must be broken before the door can be opened. This is done by admitting air, which is filtered to remove any microbes that might compromise the sterility of the load.

Many hospital autoclaves operate at about three times atmospheric pressure. To contain this, the walls of an autoclave chamber must be very thick, and to avoid accidents this 'pressure vessel' should (and in many countries must by law) be tested regularly to ensure there are no cracks that might weaken it and cause an explosion. During sterilization, these walls are exposed to steam at the same time as the load they contain. Condensation on the walls continues until the mass of metal of which they are made reaches the temperature of the steam. The large amount of water produced in this way makes the contents of the autoclave wet. Although of no consequence for unwrapped items, this is unacceptable for anything wrapped in materials through which steam must, and so water can, pass. When a package is removed from an autoclave, a wet wrapping provides a liquid channel through which bacteria can float or even actively swim and so penetrate the sterile interior.

To avoid this, most standard autoclave chambers are surrounded by hollow jackets that are kept filled with steam. If operated correctly, these keep the walls of the chamber at a temperature just below the working temperature of the autoclave. This reduces condensation during the sterilizing cycle. The jacket must not heat the chamber above the sterilizing temperature, or the steam entering it may be superheated, converting the autoclave into a much less efficient hot-air oven. At the end of a cycle, the jacket also helps to dry out the small amount of moisture that condenses in the load during sterilization. Of course, the door of an autoclave cannot easily be fitted with a steam jacket, and so some condensation takes place on the inside of this. The doors of a double-ended autoclave double this disadvantage, and they also provide extra joints through which air may leak. Double-ended autoclaves are not recommended for general use.

Although often automated, all autoclaves pass through certain stages in completing a sterilizing cycle. First, the autoclave is loaded, not too tightly, and the door is closed. Next, the air is removed. This is done by various methods, depending on the type and design of the machine. This is followed by the sterilizing phase, during which the load is raised to the predetermined temperature and held there for the required time. Next, the steam is removed and air is admitted to return the chamber to atmospheric pressure. Finally, the door is opened and the load removed.

Many standard autoclaves are fitted with controls that allow different sterilizing cycles to be employed. These may be used to sterilize delicate items at lower temperatures for longer times, or to process bottles containing liquids. In the latter case, the autoclave door must not be opened until the liquid has cooled, as a bottle containing liquid at above 100°C may explode when the pressure is reduced. Small, cheaper autoclaves without steam jackets in which steam is generated by boiling water inside the chamber are useful in some settings (outpatient departments and small dental or medical clinics, for example). These are suitable for sterilizing unwrapped instruments and other items required for immediate use. Special autoclaves are employed in pharmacies where significant amounts of liquids are sterilized, particularly if they are packed in plastic containers. Some operating departments have installed autoclaves that operate at higher temperatures to allow very short sterilizing cycles. These 'flash' or 'dropped instrument' sterilizers are sometimes used for the routine processing of items. If this is done, the cycles used should be validated as for any other autoclave.

As with hot-air ovens, the twin parameters of time and temperature are the prime physical measures of sterilizing ability in an autoclave. As temperature and pressure are connected, it is usual to measure both, preferably with an instrument that makes a permanent record. However, the quality of the steam admitted to the autoclave and the amount of residual air in the chamber during sterilization are factors that can cause failure. This may happen despite adequate exposure at a proper pressure, and the temperature record may mislead. For practical reasons, the temperature is usually measured at a point other than where it really matters, which is inside the load being sterilized. To be at its most efficient, steam must be at the 'phase boundary', that is, just saturated, neither containing water droplets (wet or supersaturated steam) nor being superheated (dry steam). This condition is difficult to measure directly, and so is left to engineers to arrange. A more common cause of failure is the presence of too much residual air in the chamber. This may happen because the air-removing system has failed, or more often, because of leaks. These are always important, but in porous load autoclaves, even an invisible hole in a door seal or at a joint between pipes may allow the entry of significant amounts of air during the vacuum phase of the cycle.

There are a number of different ways in which an autoclave may be shown to have worked correctly. Reliance may be placed on physical parameters (time, temperature and pressure), or on biological indicators, or on physical or chemical devices that change their colour or form on exposure to a certain temperature for a certain time, or on any combination of these. The choice of method or methods is the subject of a debate that sometimes gets as hot as the steam being tested!

Physical measurements are precise and objective, and the results are available immediately, and so a load can be passed as sterile at once. They suffer from the disadvantage that the measurements are recorded by instruments that must be calibrated regularly to ensure accuracy and, as noted, steam quality and air removal are important though less easily measured components of success. When physical parameters are used to monitor autoclaves, the simpler measures are backed up by a programme of extra physical tests that include a search for leaks, and the use of thermocouples to make direct measurements of the temperature achieved at various points in the chamber. This is done on a regular basis by trained operatives using special instruments. An advantage of this approach is that the accuracy of the measurements made are sufficient to plot small progressive deteriorations before they affect the efficiency of a machine. This allows corrective maintenance to be a planned activity rather than a response to a breakdown. Of course, catastrophic failure cannot be predicted, but as this is often due to the sudden development of a leak, the eventuality is covered by the daily performance of a Bowie-Dick test.

The Bowie-Dick test is a test for air removal and steam penetration, and so is only applicable to porous-load autoclaves. The test should be performed as the first run of each autoclave every working day. The pack used is placed at about the centre of an autoclave that is otherwise empty. The traditional pack is made up of up to 36 clean, dry, preferably huckaback hand-towels. Each is folded into eight thicknesses, and they are stacked until an approximate cube is formed 11–12 inches (280–305 mm) high. A piece of paper bearing a St Andrew's cross of 3M brand autoclave tape is placed between the towels at the centre of the stack. When the autoclave cycle is complete, the stack is removed and the tape examined. If the tape has changed colour evenly right across both arms of the cross, the autoclave has passed the test. A failure is indicated by the colour change being less intense at the centre than at the outside of each arm of the tape. This is due to residual air in the chamber that is compressed into a bubble at the centre of the pack, where it excludes steam and prevents sterilization. If an autoclave fails the Bowie-Dick test, it must not be used until it has been repaired. Commercial equivalents of the Bowie-Dick test pack are available.

In a biological test, the autoclave is challenged to kill something approaching a million spores of *B. stearothermophilus*. One or more paper strips impregnated with the spores enclosed in glassine envelopes or other steam-permeable containers are included inside typical packs to be autoclaved. On completion of the cycle, the strips are extracted and are cultured microbiologically to detect any spores that may have survived. Commercial kits that contain the spores and the necessary culture medium have been developed, so that the test can be carried out within the department housing the autoclave. As with any biological test, a positive control (a strip that has not been autoclaved) must be included with each batch of cultures to show that the spores were viable at the outset. The test takes at least 48 hours and, perhaps, seven days to complete. For safety, the contents of the autoclave may be stored until the test indicates that sterilization has been successful. If it is adopted, the necessity for quarantine has cost implications. A failed test requires the autoclave to be taken out of use until the fault has been found and corrected. The test can only give a negative or a positive result, so no advance warning of impending autoclave failure is provided. As it is a biological test it is poorly reproducible, though because of the degree of over-kill in an autoclave, this is not very important. It is customary to use the Bowie-Dick test in combination with biological tests.

A number of devices are available commercially that may be put inside packs during sterilization. These change their colour or some other aspect of their appearance when exposed for a certain time at a particular temperature. Once they have been validated by an independent authority, they must be used with strict compliance to their manufacturers' instructions, particularly with regard to storage conditions and shelf-life. They are generally less satisfactory than the other control methods described.

The incinerator

Fire simultaneously sterilizes and consumes what is burnt. On the face of it, incineration provides the ideal way of dealing with hospital waste which is simultaneously reduced to a negligible volume and freed of obnoxious characteristics and infectious potential. Unfortunately, this is not the whole story. Apart from the ecological damage they do (below, p. 126), incinerators have several more immediate disadvantages. If material sent for incineration contains much liquid, as it may if placentas, incontinence pads or disposable suction bottles are burnt, the process will consume significant amounts of oil or gas to achieve destruction. Hospital waste is almost certain to include a proportion, perhaps large, of plastic. Where too much dense black smoke is produced, it will be unacceptable to neighbours and clean-air inspectors alike. An invisible but more damaging by-product of the burning of plastic is hydrochloric acid, which before passing out into the atmosphere attacks the incinerator itself and shortens its life. There is concern about the small particles, perhaps including some carrying microbes, that may be swept up the chimneys by the flue gasses in simple incinerators before they can be burnt. This possibility has imposed expensive modifications in design. In many places where they are still used, these various disadvantages have led to a reduction in the volume of material dealt with by incinerators and, in some countries, restrictive or even prohibitive regulation or legislation has been introduced.

Sterilization by radiation
Cost, complexity and very stringent safety requirements surround the use of ionizing radiations (usually gamma rays) for sterilization. This has limited the practice almost completely to very large facilities dealing with disposable items, such as mass-produced syringes. Recently, smaller units have appeared that might be suitable for use in hospitals. If these prove cost-effective, they will require most careful monitoring by people who know enough about the physics of radiation to ensure both safety and sterilizing efficiency.

Chemical sterilization
Although other chemicals (notably formaldehyde) have been used in sterilizing processes, only ethylene oxide (EO) is in common use for medical purposes.

EO is a non-corrosive, extremely penetrating, highly effective sterilizing agent. Unfortunately, it is flammable and explosive when mixed with air at certain concentrations, and it is irritant, toxic, mutagenic and carcinogenic. It is colourless and remains odourless at concentrations well above those that are toxic. Unless sensitive automatic detecting devices are fitted in places where the gas is used, personnel may be exposed to danger without being aware of it. Personal monitors may also be worn. As concern has grown in many countries about the possible toxic effects of EO, the maximum permissible level to which workers can be exposed has fallen progressively.

Successful sterilization with EO is dependant on even more factors than is the case with steam under pressure. Time, temperature, humidity, pressure and gas concentrations are all important. Some machines work at increased pressure, mixing the EO with an inert gas, such as carbon dioxide or the even more ecologically unfriendly chlorofluorocarbon (CFC). This reduces the risk of explosion, but increases the likelihood of leaks. Other machines work at sub-atmospheric pressure. Different manufacturers use different sterilizing cycles.

Wrapped items that have been sterilized in EO require lengthy aeration to free them of residual gas before they are used. To reduce the exposure of staff when unloading the machine, this may be carried out initially for up to 18 hours inside the sterilizing chamber itself. Following this, further aeration is required which varies with the material concerned (rubber, silicone and polyvinyl chloride take longer) and the temperature at which the process is carried out. Even at a high temperature (55°C), 12 hours is necessary.

Because many of the factors on which the production of sterility depend are difficult to measure, EO machines are monitored biologically. In this case, spores of *B. subtilis* may be employed. The procedure is as described for steam sterilizers, though as there is no other control spore strips should be exposed in each cycle. One may suffice in a small sterilizer, though several are needed when monitoring very large machines. If items with long, narrow lumens are to be sterilized, a strip should be placed at the most distal or difficult point or, if this is impossible, a special test piece is used (Line and Pickerill, 1973), or one may be constructed locally by attaching a narrow tube to the cap of a small bottle in which the spore strip is placed. The spores are usually retrieved for culture after the preliminary aeration in the sterilizer chamber is complete. The need to quarantine packs until a negative spore culture is recorded has cost implications. Many of the items sterilized by EO are expensive, and so may not be available in such numbers as to allow them to be out of use for the long period necessary. Of course, part of the culture time is occupied by the aeration phase.

Although all sterilization processes should be supervised by specially trained personnel, this is particularly true in the case of EO machines. The number of items for which EO sterilization is an absolute requirement is small, and many of the things for which it is more often used can be made microbiologically safe by other methods.

EO machines are expensive, potentially dangerous and have high running costs. They should not be installed without careful thought.

Disinfecting methods

Disinfecting methods have a very broad spectrum of efficacy. At one end are the weaker methods with such low general toxicity that they can be used on or in living tissue. At the other are very powerful or toxic agents that can only be applied to 'things'. In practice, these may often produce sterility, but this cannot be guaranteed, and so they are included here. Although neither sterilization nor disinfection are instantaneous, the time element is more important with disinfection. Most sterilizers are fitted with timing devices so they cannot be opened prematurely: indeed, it might be fatally dangerous for the operator to do so. Disinfection takes longer, sometimes much longer. As the process is usually under the control of the person applying it, natural impatience may cut the time of application to the point that even disinfection is not achieved. The great importance of thorough cleaning before items are disinfected is stressed again.

Heat

The application of heat to produce disinfection is by the use of hot water, or steam. Steam at atmospheric pressure (about 100°C) applied in a steamer is now rarely used outside laboratories, but specially designed, low-temperature steam autoclaves that operate at sub-atmospheric pressure (say 355 mm of mercury and 80°C) are available (Alder *et al.*, 1971). These produce a very high order of disinfection in wrapped items that might be damaged by higher temperatures. If formaldehyde is added to this process, sterility can be achieved. Technical difficulties still need to be overcome before the low-temperature steam and formaldehyde process is generally accepted. It would be an attractive alternative to EO not least because the human nose can detect formaldehyde at levels below that at which toxicity is thought to be a problem.

Boiling water is an extremely efficient, high-level disinfecting agent. It fails to kill only a few resistant spores of kinds almost never found on clean surfaces. It was given a bad press during the campaign that accompanied the transfer of instrument preparation from hospital wards to central supply organizations. It is unlikely that any clean instrument that was boiled for not less than five minutes ever caused an infection. The argument that instrument 'boilers' were dangerous to staff who are notorious for their use of boiling water for making tea or coffee is not easily sustained. The main problem with boilers was that they were abused by being overfilled by multiple users, so that no one knew if an item had been in water (that may have ceased to boil) for 30 seconds or three hours. Another problem was how to disinfect the notorious Cheatle forceps with which items were removed from the boiler. When all is said and done, however, it is well to remember that in an emergency, properly timed exposure to water that is really boiling is a better, quicker, cheaper, more readily available and more convenient near-sterilizing method than any other.

For items that cannot be boiled, pasteurization may be carried out in water at temperatures between 60°C and 90°C for times varying with temperature from a few seconds to an hour. This is again a very effective disinfecting agent. After all, properly pasteurized milk is very safe to drink.

Ultraviolet light

Short-wavelength uV light can kill or inactivate microbes. Sunlight is quite good as a disinfecting agent. Provided artificial uV sources contain sufficient short-wavelength uV radiation, they are effective antimicrobially, if nothing obstructs it. Short-wavelength uV light does not penetrate far into liquids, and it is stopped by a thin layer of dust or other dirt on the glass of the source lamp. As a lamp ages, the wavelength of the light it emits lengthens, and so although the lamp appears to be operating normally, it may be deficient in antimicrobial activity. Special apparatus is required to detect this gradual loss of efficiency. Experiments have been performed in the use of uV radiation to treat the air in occupied spaces, to reduce infections. This approach has failed to reduce respiratory infections in schools, or to have much influence on surgical infections (Chapter 4, p. 72). Another application has been in the production of near-sterile water for clinical purposes. With a new lamp and clean surfaces, this works quite well, but deterioration due to the factors mentioned above results in a loss of efficiency that will pass unnoticed unless regular monitoring is carried out.

Disinfectants and antiseptics

Bad smells are very often a by-product of bacterial putrefaction. For this reason, the human nose can detect the presence of certain kinds of bacteria, and this led to the use of disinfectants before microbes were discovered. Certain chemicals were found to control smells, and because smells were associated with disease, they were also used to try to control infection. Chlorine and carbolic acid were employed in this way well over 100 years ago, and are still used in the form of hypochlorite and phenolic disinfectants. A number of other chemicals have joined them. It is notable that a direct relationship exists between the degree of toxicity of a disinfectant to man, and its general ability to kill or inactivate microbes. Very powerful disinfectants are extremely toxic to all living matter, while disinfectants (antiseptics) that can safely be used on skin or mucous membranes are significantly weaker, and are only effective against certain classes or types of microbe. Some more hardy bacteria are able to grow in solutions of weak disinfectants and have caused infections in patients on whom supposedly 'sterile' antiseptics have been used. Weak disinfectants may not even disinfect themselves.

Disinfectants, particularly these weaker ones, are best supplied sterile, in single-use containers. If this is not possible, disinfectant concentrates may be stored in bottles that are reopened occasionally with fair safety, but once a disinfectant has been diluted, any residue should be discarded immediately after use or at the most after an hour or two. Bottles of stock disinfectants should never be 'topped up', but fresh, clean, preferably sterile bottles should be used each time. Some disinfectants are inactivated by cork, soap, hard water, plastics or rubber. Products bought from reputable manufacturers will include warnings about this in their literature.

All disinfectants attack organic matter more or less indiscriminately, and are used up in doing so. If microbes are enmeshed in a large amount of dirt, a disinfectant applied to the mixture may be exhausted before all the microbes are killed or, indeed, before it has penetrated much below the surface. This is why objects to be disinfected should whenever possible be cleaned beforehand. When this is not possible, more concentrated preparations of disinfectants may be used, often described in the accompanying literature as being appropriate for 'dirty' situations.

Because of wide variations in availability and in national regulations and prejudices, only general comments are made here about individual disinfectants. Each hospital should have its own disinfectant policy, prepared by the ICT or ICC. It is an expensive mistake to provide a large range of different disinfectant products to cater for a multitude of individual preferences. It is important to note that many of the most advanced hospitals have abandoned the use of disinfectants in environmental cleaning, replacing them with a simple detergent in water (Chapter 7, p. 156).

Most hospitals will find that one disinfectant representing each of the five general classes of disinfectants and antiseptics that follow will be sufficient for their needs, though in certain cases more than one formulation of a particular product will be required.

1. A powerful general-purpose agent for use in disinfecting accidental spills of potentially infected body fluids, etc. This must be active against all microbes. Chlorine as hypochlorite is most commonly used for this. It should be purchased in the most concentrated form available commercially (10% available chlorine, or 100000 parts per million (ppm). Note that one quite widely used and expensive form is supplied at only 1% or 10000 ppm). Hypochlorite is used at 1% (10000 ppm) for spills, 0.1% (1000 ppm) for general environmental disinfection, and may be used at 0.001% (100 ppm) for the disinfection of teats and other equipment associated with infant feeding. Solution tablets of sodium dichloroisocyanurate are an alternative, initially more expensive, but more convenient and less wasteful form of hypochlorite. They are available from a variety of commercial sources. Hypochlorite is a highly effective disinfectant, but may corrode metal and damage plastics, rubber and fabrics. It is unsuitable for most metal instruments, but is non-toxic at low concentrations, and so it may be used for catering equipment. Of course, it is widely used at concentrations of 5 ppm or less to make drinking water and the water in swimming pools microbiologically safe. Note that chlorine has been used as a poison gas in war. Although it would not be easy to generate significant amounts of the gas from products designed for disinfectant use, they should be treated with respect, and not employed in enclosed, poorly ventilated spaces.

2. Glutaraldehyde, kinder to metal and plastics than hypochlorite, is available in various forms from several commercial sources. Its principal use is to disinfect endoscopes. It is important to pay particular attention to the literature provided by the manufacturers of both the disinfectant and the endoscope, and to heed the advice of various professional bodies in the field. Although sometimes described as a sterilant, it is usually applied for too short a time to achieve sterilization. While most bacteria are killed in 2 minutes, HIV and the hepatitis B virus may take 10–30 minutes, tubercle bacilli 60 minutes and spores 3–10 hours. Glutaraldehyde is toxic, irritant and allergenic. Gloves must be worn when handling it, tanks of it require to be covered, and rooms where it is used need to be well ventilated. Of course, an instrument soaked in it must be thoroughly rinsed in sterile water before it is used.

   Special equipment has been devised and is commercially available for the disinfection of endoscopes with glutaraldehyde. Fluids are actively pumped through the various endoscopic channels, and so the process is quite efficient. If endoscopes are simply soaked in the various fluids, two points require attention. First, if instruments are wet when immersed in the glutaraldehyde solution, significant dilution of the disinfectant may result as successive instruments are treated. Secondly, care must be taken to ensure that the disinfectant and rinsing solutions reach into all parts of the apparatus. In particular, there must be no bubbles in narrow channels. The chances of this are reduced if instruments are immersed vertically in tall tanks rather than being laid flat in trays.

3. Phenolics may be used for environmental disinfection in situations in which bacterial pathogens are to be attacked, and hypochlorite is inappropriate. A large range of 'clear soluble phenolics' is available from commercial sources.

4. Alcohol (ethyl alcohol, sometimes called spirit, or isopropyl alcohol) diluted in water to 70% is a very effective disinfectant. It is particularly useful because it evaporates, and so does not have to be washed off after disinfection, and surfaces are left dry. Alcohol does not kill spores, but is active against all other microbes. It can be used on intact skin where it is the best disinfectant for general use, either on its own or in combination with a residual disinfectant to prolong the effect. It can be distributed in liquid form, or impregnated into paper tissues packed individually or multiply. These are useful when disinfecting skin or other surfaces. Alcohol is flammable.

5. There are a number of skin and tissue antiseptics, of which povidone iodine and chlorhexidine are the most widely used. Either may be employed in aqueous solution for use on mucous membranes or exposed tissues. Combined with a detergent they may be used as antiseptic surgical scrubs or for cleaning dirty wounds. Formulated with alcohol they become useful skin disinfectants or they may be incorporated in an ointment. Povidone iodine has a broad antimicrobial spectrum, though its action is rather slow, particularly against spores. Chlorhexidine is more active against Gram-positive than Gram-negative bacteria, but has no activity against tubercle bacilli or spores. It is effective against fungi and some viruses, including HIV.

Antimicrobial drugs

The history of the successful use of chemicals in infections began in 1619, with the first record of the treatment of malaria with cinchona bark (quinine) in Peru. At about the same time, ipecacuanha root (emetine) was found to be useful in the treatment of what is now known to be the amoebic variety of dysentery. These alkaloids were joined later by the organic arsenicals for syphilis, and in 1909 by Erlich's salvarsan for protozoal infections. A major advance came in

1935 when the first true antibacterial agent, prontosil (the original sulphonamide), was introduced. In 1929, Fleming discovered the first antibiotic, penicillin, though this was not used therapeutically until the early 1940s. Substances produced by one microbe that damage or destroy others at high dilution were called **antibiotics**, and their use in medicine for the treatment of infections was called **antibiotic therapy**. Similar drugs that were synthesized by chemical means were called **chemotherapeutic agents**, and their use was **chemotherapy**.

Since the early days, many new chemotherapeutic drugs have been produced, and a large number of antibiotics have been discovered. At the same time, the nomenclature has become confused. Some drugs that were originally antibiotics are now produced by chemical synthesis (for instance, chloramphenicol), and so they have changed into chemotherapeutic agents. Several drugs (ampicillin, for example) are made by synthetic alteration of an antibiotic precursor, and so are hybrids. More recently, a number of compounds introduced for the treatment of malignant diseases have been called chemotherapeutic agents. To avoid confusion, the term **antimicrobial drug** is now used to cover all antimicrobial chemotherapeutic agents and antibiotics.

The antimicrobials are unique among drugs, as they are required to act in the presence of two separate living organisms, to damage or destroy one while so far as possible leaving the other unharmed. Many that are active against bacteria can do no more than stop them multiplying (bacteriostatic agents), and so depend on the normal defensive mechanisms of the body to remove residual microbes. Bactericidal antimicrobial drugs do kill bacteria, but only when they are actively multiplying. Any large population of bacteria contain a proportion that are 'resting' (in a stationary phase of growth), and so even the bactericidal drugs need the help of the normal defences of the body to clear away a mass of infecting microbes.

As noted, most antimicrobial agents originated as the products of microbes themselves. For millenia, microbes have used antimicrobials as weapons in their struggle to survive and be successful among their neighbours. In any war, the appearance of a new weapon on one side leads to the invention of counter-measures on the other. Bacteria soon learnt how to defend themselves when they were attacked by a fungus or another bacterium that knew how to make antimicrobials. There was nothing new about antimicrobials when the human race discovered them, and this explains why when an antimicrobial drug is used for the first time it has at best a temporary advantage. This lasts until the mechanisms developed by microbes over many thousands of years to counter antimicrobial attack are rearranged to deal with the new threat. Perversely, the resistant microbes that then appear are encouraged as the drug clears a space for them among their sensitive neighbours.

No antimicrobial drug is active against all microbes. Each anti-bacterial, antiviral or antiprotozoal drug has a 'spectrum' of activity, which describes the range of bacteria, viruses or protozoa that are damaged or killed by it. Some antimicrobials have a narrow spectrum, and so are active against just a few kinds of microbe, while others have a broader spectrum. When treating an infection due to a microbe that has been identified, it is preferable to use a narrow-spectrum drug to attack it. In this way, harmless members of the body's normal flora are not removed unnecessarily, or put under selective pressure to become resistant. If this is done coherently as a result of a policy decision in a hospital, the development of antimicrobial resistance is delayed, and so far as possible kept under control.

Hospitals in which broad-spectrum antimicrobials are routine first choices quickly develop a population of multi-resistant hospital strains of bacteria. Regrettably, such hospitals are also more likely to be places where antimicrobials are prescribed very freely for the least, and too often inappropriate, indication. Patients suffer as a result because any real infections are then more difficult to treat. More expensive and sometimes more toxic drugs have to be used when simpler drugs would otherwise have sufficed. ICTs and ICCs have a responsibility to press for the responsible use of antimicrobial drugs. The target ought to be a rational 'antimicrobial policy' tailored to the needs of each hospital or group of hospitals.

REUSING DISPOSABLES

The title of this section is a contradiction. Disposable medical equipment is made to be used once, then thrown away. Manufacturers and the medical authorities in some richer countries (for different reasons, we hope) are quick to point out that items meant for single use cannot be guaranteed to work properly or, indeed, may fail structurally if used more than once, and that it may be difficult or impossible to clean and, if necessary, resterilize them between uses. If the apparatus has a volumetric function, they say that accuracy may be lost. Finally, they highlight the fact that if an accident occurs as the result of reusing a disposable, the fault lies with the user, who must bear the consequences, including the cost of any litigation.

As medicine has become more technical, the equipment necessary to it has extended enormously in range and complexity. At one time, much of it was made to be reused. A revolution followed the appearance of improved plastics and of the skills needed to manipulate them. Commercial and other pressures led to cost-effectiveness studies that showed that money could be saved by replacing some reusable equipment with single-use disposable items made of plastic. These studies may have left out certain costs, such as that of providing the extended facilities required to transport or store the greater volume of disposables, or the cost of getting rid of them after use. They certainly took no account of the damage their disposal has done and is still doing to incinerators or to the environment (below, p. 126). Today new forms of equipment are often disposable from the outset. Most of it is attractive to look at and pleasant to handle, but the cost of it is now an important part of health-care budgets. Even in the richest countries, some of the more expensive 'single-use' items, such as cardiac catheters, pacemakers and haemodialysis coils, are recycled. In the poorest countries, 'disposable' syringes may be reused up to 40 times. In the middle, a wide range of equipment is reprocessed, including items such as eye shields, oxygen masks, airways, anaesthetic tubing, tracheostomy and endotracheal tubes and fetal scalp electrodes. It is clear that a wide gap exists between what the manufacturers would like and what really happens.

If a hospital decides to reuse single use items, the decision should be made consciously in each case, with full consultation that should include the ICC. Each step of the procedure necessary to recycling, including cleaning, examination for structural integrity and, if appropriate, testing for function, the type of any packaging required and the method used for sterilization or disinfection should be defined and written down. The work should be supervised by a responsible person, and may be integrated into hospital sterilizing and disinfecting units (Chapter 7, p. 146).

As with any disinfection or sterilization process, the preliminary wash is of vital importance. This is particularly true of tubes, more so if they are long and thin, and might contain blood that has clotted. It may be necessary to devise a special flushing system in these cases, and to show that the tube is fully patent before it is processed any further. The final flush, at least for items used parenterally, should be with distilled water. Washing is followed by drying, perhaps with warm air but, in any case, in an atmosphere free at least of larger particles of dust. A competent engineer can adapt electric hair driers and simple air filters for this purpose.

The options for sterilization or disinfection include autoclaving, ethylene oxide, low temperature steam, hot-water pasteurization and exposure to disinfectants, of which glutaraldehyde, formaldehyde, alcohol and hypochlorite have most commonly been used (above, p. 117). Among the plastics, polystyrene will barely stand up to pasteurization, though with care PVC (vinyl) will. Polypropylene, PTFE, and epoxy and silicone resins will all withstand autoclaving. For less critical items that will only come into contact with non-sterile mucous membranes, pasteurization is an adequate process. Liquid chemicals should be used only when there is no alternative.

Accidents resulting from the reuse of single-use equipment are not in evidence. Provided recycling is performed responsibly, there is no reason why it should add perceptibly to the risks already inherent in modern medical treatment. Much of the population of the world has no access to modern medicine, which is rationed even in the richest countries. If the money saved by recycling disposables is used to help people who would otherwise be deprived of medical care, then so be it.

WASTE AND ITS DISPOSAL

It is a common human perception that waste is at least potentially and often actually offensive, and that it is a health hazard. This perception is highlighted when the waste arises in a hospital. Media reports of the finding of such things as used syringes or even human tissues in refuse tips or washed up on beaches has made this a major public issue. Hospital administrators must pay proper attention to the disposal of their waste, or they risk adverse publicity and, perhaps, public humiliation.

As often happens, public perception has linked the unaesthetic with the hazardous. With certain specific exceptions, the vast mass of hospital waste is certainly no more dangerous than that generated in ordinary households. In hospitals, wet food waste (with its potential for supporting bacterial multiplication) is usually separated from the inherently much safer dry waste, and so what emerges for disposal is often less objectionable in a microbiological sense than household waste. Even if it were not so, the distinction between a reservoir and a source of infection must be made in this case (Chapter 2, p. 28). Short of physically rolling about in rubbish, it is difficult to see how any microbes it may contain could cause an infection. With the important exception of penetrating injuries due to bloodstained sharp objects and exposure to excrement, instances of infection arising from exposure to rubbish, either from hospitals or the rest of the community, are not evident.

Hospital waste needs to be categorized into different classes if the most stringent (and expensive) disposal procedures are not to be applied to the whole of it. The 'clinical waste' for which special disposal methods are necessary may not exceed 10% of the total.

Table 5.3 Categories of waste that arise in hospitals

Categories of waste	Disposal method
1. Excremental and other liquid waste	Water carried sewage system, if available (see below)
2. Domestic rubbish (trash): (a) used paper, plastic, etc. (b) catering department waste	Same method as used in the surrounding community for household or food waste with recycling wherever possible
3. Clinical waste: (a) offensive or microbially hazardous waste* (b) human tissue (c) microbially hazardous laboratory waste, AFTER autoclaving in house	Incineration or such other methods as are approved by national regulatory bodies
(d) sharp objects	Direct disposal into special 'sharps container' (see below). When full this is incinerated or dealt with as above
(e) residues of certain particularly toxic drugs or radioactive materials	As required by national regulatory bodies
(f) other waste (confidential documents, pharmaceuticals, flammable materials, etc.)	May be incinerated, or as determined locally

*Used dressings, incontinence pads, disposable suction bottles, disposable sputum pots, etc.

If discipline is imposed on what constitutes dangerous waste, the proportion might be reduced still further. Waste is classified in Table 5.3, where for completeness excremental waste (faeces and urine) is included.

In places where a public, water-carried sewage system is not available, a considerable problem may arise with the disposal of faeces and urine. If disposal can be arranged by water carriage into properly designed and maintained private sewage systems or septic tanks, then the situation is retrieved. However, this is not always possible and, unfortunately, it is precisely in these places that diseases with a faecal-oral route of transmission may be much more common. Here patients with enteric fever (typhoid or paratyphoid), dysentery, cholera or some forms of hepatitis are often found in hospitals. Unless some hygienic method of disposal of faeces and urine can be devised, such patients are a hazard to other patients, to staff and to the community round the hospital. The addition of a disinfectant to bedpans is not a complete answer, for two reasons. First, the amount of disinfectant is unlikely to be sufficient to do what is necessary and, secondly, the toxic phenolic disinfectants commonly used contaminate the environment, and may find their way back into drinking water.

Special containers for the disposal of sharp objects ('sharps containers') are necessary because of the unacceptably high incidence of accidents to hospital employees. In many cases, these have suffered needle-stick and other injuries from the growing number of disposable sharp objects when handling bags of ordinary waste into which they were placed. Infection with hepatitis B has followed such accidents, and the possibility of HIV infection is now an extra hazard. Sharps containers need to be rigid and waterproof, and made of a material that cannot easily be penetrated by, for instance, a hypodermic needle. Ideally, the top opening should be arranged so that once inserted, an object cannot be removed or escape if the container is upset. When full, it should be possible to close this opening in a positive fashion for safe disposal (Gwyther, 1990).

In using sharps containers, opinions differ on whether, for instance, a syringe should be discarded with the needle attached, or if the needle should be put into the container on its own and the syringe discarded elsewhere. Some containers are equipped with key-holes into which the hub of a needle can be fitted, to allow it to be twisted off so that it falls inside without risk to the hands of the operator. The argument turns largely on the cost of sharps containers, and the speed with which they are filled. In places where the cost of special sharps containers is prohibitive, an alternative is to use the plastic containers in which liquids (disinfectants, for instance) are supplied to the hospital. In any case, containers should not be filled right to the top. If something is forced into an already over-filled container, somewhere a needle may be pushed through the side of it. Sharps containers do not need to be discarded on some regular basis, but only when they are sufficiently full.

For a long time, incineration was seen as the ideal way to dispose of, at least, the clinical category of waste, and sometimes all of it. This is no longer universally true, and the increasing proportion of disposable plastic used in hospitals is one of the chief problems. This has significantly increased the volume of waste while only marginally increasing its weight. At one time, when an incinerator was to be installed its size was determined by the weight of material to be burnt rather than its volume, and so many are now too small.

This is not all. When plastic is burnt it tends to produce dense black smoke, and its by-products are carbon dioxide, a significant amount of hydrochloric acid and small amounts of other very toxic compounds. The smoke is unacceptable to communities with Clean Air Acts, the carbon dioxide contributes to the greenhouse effect, the acid eats away the inside of the incinerator and becomes acid rain, and the toxins are very environmentally unfriendly. Some of these problems may be overcome by using more sophisticated and expensive incinerators, but the international concern for the environment has already led some countries to produce legislation or regulations that effectively prevent their use. This attitude is likely to spread. Alternative methods for rendering clinical waste both safe and aesthetically acceptable are beginning to appear, but they are expensive, depend on complex machinery that might break down, and produce a bulky end product that still has to be disposed of.

The usual alternative to incineration is landfill. For overpopulated or environmentally very conscious countries, it has become increasingly difficult to find sites where this is socially or ecologically acceptable. Perhaps more seriously there is growing concern about the leakage of toxic materials from these dumps. In some cases, these already have reached drinking water, and in other cases it is feared they might do so some time in the future. Greenhouse gases and compounds that destroy ozone escape into the air as some kinds of rubbish undergoes microbial degradation.

The problems that afflict hospitals when they try to dispose of their waste is no more than a rather acute reflection of a difficulty that increasingly involves the whole human race. The 'effluent society' that inhabits the more affluent parts of the globe is already a cliché, but it cannot be long before we are forced to do something about it. Pressure to do so comes from three sides. First is the growing problem of what to do with the volume of waste already being produced. Secondly, as the population of the world expands, the 'effluent' group gets larger and its waste more voluminous and, incidentally, the difference between the 'haves' and 'havenots' grows more stark. Thirdly is the finite nature of the earth's resources. In the case of disposable plastics, hydrocarbons that have taken millions of years to form are converted into an item that is used once and then is either burnt (so in a few weeks is converted back into carbon dioxide), or put into a hole in the ground where it is likely to remain intact for centuries. Exhaustion of the earth's store of hydrocarbons or global warming or both will put an end to this profligacy if we do not do something about it. As a first step, manufacturers ought to be persuaded to stop wrapping items in packages that are often many times larger than they need be, and perhaps heavier than the item itself. They should also recycle their packaging and other plastic materials. Hospitals may be driven to reverse the move towards making everything disposable, and they should be active in the campaign to recycle as much as possible. The point at which it would be cheaper to revert to reusable glass syringes may not be far away.

The ICC or whatever body is appointed for the purpose in each hospital ought to take these factors into account as they produce new or modify existing waste disposal policies. At the same time, the supplies organization should develop an environmental conscience and press manufacturers to remove the rubbish they generate. So far as waste is concerned, it is necessary to decide on the number of categories to be identified, and arrange for the supply of suitable bags in an equivalent number of distinctive colours to pack it in. Then, taking account of local conditions and probably of existing regulations, the method of disposal is chosen. Incineration at the hospital or at a distant shared site are options. When a distant site or landfill is to be used, a secure means of transport as well as site security are required. In either case, vermin-proof and child-proof storage is needed wherever bags of waste are stored prior to disposal.

One of the most important parts of the whole system is a training programme designed so that all members of staff know and understand the hospital policy, and are motivated to adhere to it. Finally, the system ought to be monitored actively to correct errors before these become matters of public concern.

FURTHER READING

Ayliffe, G. A. J. (1988) Equipment-related infection risks. *J. Hosp. Infect.*, **11** (Supplement), 279–84.

Ayliffe, G. A. J., Coates, D. and Hoffman, P. N. (1984) *Chemical Disinfection in Hospitals*. Public Health Laboratory Service, London.

Babb, J. R. (1988) Methods of reprocessing complex medical equipment. *J. Hosp. Infect.*, **11** (Supplement), 285–91.

Gardner, J. F. and Peel, M. M. (1986) *Introduction to Sterilization and Disinfection*. Churchill Livingstone, Melbourne.

Kolmos, H. J. (1983) A clinical and bacteriological evaluation of a re-use system for disposable haemodyalisers. *J. Hosp. Infect.*, **4**, 269–78.

REFERENCES

Albert, R. K. and Condie, F. C. (1981) Hand-washing patterns in medical intensive-care units. *New Eng. J. Med.*, **304**, 1465–6.

Alder, V. G., Gingell, J. C. and Mitchell, J. P. (1971) Disinfection of cystoscopes by subatmospheric steam and steam and formaldehyde at 80°C. *Brit. Med. J.*, **ii**, 677–80.

Ayliffe, G. A. J., Babb, J. R., Taylor, L. *et al.* (1979) A unit for source and protective isolation in a general hospital. *Brit. Med. J.*, **ii**, 461–5.

Centers for Disease Control (1988) Update: universal precautions for prevention of transmission of human immunodeficiency virus, hepatitis B virus, and other bloodborne pathogens in health care settings. *MMWR*, **37**, 377–88.

Duguid, J. P. (1946) The size and duration of air carriage of respiratory droplets and droplet nuclei. *J. Hyg., Camb.*, **44**, 471–9.

Garner, J. S. and Simmons, B. P. (1983) CDC guidelines for isolation precautions in hospitals. *Infect. Control*, **4**, 245–325.

Garner, J. S. and Simmons, B. P. (1986) Isolation precautions, in *Hospital Infections*, 2nd edn, (eds J. V. Bennett and P. S. Brachman) Little Brown, Boston, pp. 143–50.

Gillespie, W. A., Alder, V. G., Ayliffe, G. A. J. *et al.* (1959) Staphylococcal cross-infection in surgery. Effects of some preventive measures. *Lancet*, **ii**, 781–4.

Gwyther, J. (1990) Sharps disposal containers and their use. *J. Hosp. Infect.*, **15**, 287–94.

Howells, C. H. L. and Young, H. B. (1966) A study of completely undressed surgical wounds. *Brit. J. Surg.*, **53**, 436–9.

Jarvis, J. D., Wynne, C. D., Enwright, L. *et al.* (1979) Handwashing and antiseptic-containing soaps in hospital. *J. Clin. Path.*, **32**, 732–7.

Kelsey, J. C. (1972) The myth of surgical sterility. *Lancet*, **ii**, 1301–3.

Kurtz, J. B. and Boxall, J. (1976) A partial substitute for hand washing. *Nursing Times*, **72**, 332–3.

Line, S. J. and Pickerill, J. K. (1973) Testing a steam formaldehyde sterilizer for gas penetration efficiency. *J. Clin. Path.*, **26**, 716–20.

Lynch, P., Jackson, M. M., Cummings, M. J. *et al.* (1987) Rethinking the role of isolation practices in the prevention of nosocomial infections. *Ann. Int. Med.*, **107**, 243–6.

Mathews, J. A. and Newsom, S. W. B. (1987) Hot air electric hand driers compared with paper towels for potential spread of airborne bacteria. *J. Hosp. Infect.*, **9**, 85–8.

Meers, P. D. and Leong, K. Y. (1989) Hot-air hand driers. *J. Hosp. Infect.*, **14**, 169–71.

Meers, P. D. and Leong, K. Y. (1990) The impact of methicillin- and aminoglycoside-resistant *Staphylococcus aureus* on the pattern of hospital-acquired infections in an acute hospital. *J. Hosp. Infect.*, **16**, 231–9.

Ojajarvi, J., Makela, P. and Rantasalo, I. (1977) Failure of hand disinfection with frequent hand-washing: a need for prolonged field studies. *J. Hyg., Camb.*, **79**, 107–19.

Orr, N. W. M. (1981) Is a mask necessary in the operating theatre? *Ann. Roy. Coll. Surg., Eng.*, **63**, 390–1.

Preston, G. A., Larson, E. and Stamm, W. E. (1981) The effect of private isolation rooms on patient care practices, colonization and infection in an intensive care unit. *Amer. J. Med.*, **70**, 641–5.

Reybrouck, G. (1986) Handwashing and hand disinfection. *J. Hosp. Infect.*, **8**, 5–23.

Ritter, M. A., Eitzen, H., French, M. L. V. *et al.* (1975) The operating room environment as affected by people and the surgical face mask. *Clin. Orth. and Related Res.*, **111**, 147–50.

Turner, M. J., Crowley, P. and MacDonald, D. (1984) The unmasking of delivery room routine. *J. Obs. and Gynaecol.*, **4**, 188–90.

Chapter 6

Special Environments

OPERATING DEPARTMENTS

Many of the things done to prevent surgical sepsis were originally introduced intuitively, or by extension from inadequate or misinterpreted data (see Chapters 4, p. 64), 5 (p. 98) and (p. 102)). Operating departments (ODs) are places where something called asepsis is practiced, amid much ritual.

The two major English-language dictionaries define sepsis as a toxic condition resulting from the multiplication of pathogenic bacteria and their products in the region of an infection, or as a state of poisoning of the tissues or blood stream caused by bacteria. Infection results from an interaction between two living things. If asepsis is the absence of sepsis, it follows that something inanimate or abstract cannot be 'aseptic'. Yet this extension to the meaning of the word is found in medical dictionaries. When Lister invented antiseptic surgery he imagined an attack on what he thought were the airborne causes of sepsis. As he was trying to prevent sepsis, his use of the term 'antisepsis' was correct. When surgery evolved to become aseptic the word acquired a new meaning. Aseptic surgery could accurately describe an ideal form of surgery free from infection. In fact, it was used to describe surgery or other activities performed in the (always imaginary) absence of microbes.

Although this usage is well established, it is necessary to point to the confusion it has caused. In its broad sense, the word is as difficult to define as is sterility (Chapter 5, p. 106), with the added need to decide if something is aseptic if it is contaminated with dead, though perhaps still toxic, bacteria. To highlight the problem, imagine a nurse shedding some 2000 bacteria-carrying skin squames every minute (Chapter 2, p. 30) wiping away or covering up a few hundred bacteria on a surface to prepare an 'aseptic field' to perform an 'aseptic procedure' on a patient with an infected (septic) wound. Meanwhile, both nurse and patient are home to a normal flora of some 10^{15} (1 and

15 zeros) bacteria. Even in its incorrect sense, the only truly aseptic technique would be one carried out inside an enclosure completely free of microbes in which one sterile robot operated on another. The word is so full of inconsistencies that it is meaningless. It is not suprising that such a conveniently imprecise term has become a vehicle for woolly thinking and rhetoric.

With modern technology it is (expensively) possible to achieve sterility in all parts of the environment surrounding the tissues of a patient exposed during surgery. It is inconvenient that neither these tissues nor the bodies of the patient and staff present in the OR can be sterilized. Virtually all the bacteria present in the air or on surfaces in ORs are derived from the skin of its occupants. Bacteria are shed continuously from skin (Chapter 2, p. 30), aided by movement and rubbing of clothes, and at an increased rate for some time after bathing or washing the hands (Speers *et al.*, 1965; Meers and Yeo, 1978). Normal theatre garb is no more, and may be less of a barrier to the escape of these bacteria than normal clothing (Bethune *et al.*, 1965; May and Pomeroy, 1973; Dankert *et al.*, 1979; Laufman *et al.*, 1980). After a short time, theatre dress is as prolific a source of microbes as were the outdoor clothes recently removed, or possibly more so if the person has just taken a shower. There is no **microbiological** reason for requiring theatre staff to change their clothes or for the wearing of conventional operating room garb.

For the same reason, there is no microbiological reason to distinguish between members of staff who perform 'clean' and 'dirty' tasks. Everyone carries a similar load of microbes and unless they are enclosed in an uncomfortable, all-enveloping suit made of impervious material and wear a space-style helmet, all share the habit of shedding them into their surroundings. In numerical terms, a dirty object handled with reasonable care is most unlikely to create more environmental contamination than that generated at the same time by the skin of the person performing the task. Of course, some individuals are more active disseminators of bacteria, and this becomes important if the source is an infected condition, because the large number of bacteria released are also more pathogenic (Chapter 2, p. 31).

Microbes are effectively immobile, and so depend on other agencies to carry them about. In ORs just as in any occupied building, the most important agencies are human beings, and direct contact between them the best way of effecting transfer. Transfer through the environment is very inefficient, and for most microbes the environment is hostile. Dry dust contains few bacteria, and the longer it has lain, the fewer that remain. Really heavily contaminated inanimate environmental items (a suction bottle containing pus for instance) are rare. Provided such items are securely enclosed in sealed containers or placed inside an impervious wrapper and are correctly disposed of, they pose no threat. There is no microbiological reason why contaminated and non-contaminated items or so called 'clean' and 'dirty' people should not pass each other in the same corridor. The provision of 'clean' and 'dirty' corridors in operating departments has no microbiological justification.

Transfer zones for the passage of patients, goods and staff into and out of operating departments are required for functional rather than microbiological reasons. People are the main source of bacteria, and so the number of people admitted to the department (and their activity) should be kept to a minimum. This requires discipline. Transfer zones help to impose this. It is incorrect to think the outside of a department is more heavily contaminated than the inside, and there is no evidence that sticky mats or lines painted on the floor have any microbiological value. The same reasoning means that the transfer of patients required by the two-trolley system is unnecessary (Lewis *et al.*, 1990).

The ventilation of ORs attracts a good deal of attention. There are three reasons for it. These are first, the comfort of staff and the physiological well-being of patients; secondly, the removal of flammable, explosive or toxic anaesthetic gases and, thirdly, the control of airborne microbes. Although not of direct microbiological concern, it is of interest to note that the dissipation of toxic gases by simple ventilation (the method still used for microbes) has proved inadequate. Special scavenging systems are now applied to the point at which they are released. The microbiological equivalent of this is to remove bacteria released by the body by enclosing it in the exhaust-ventilated, hooded suit employed by some orthopaedic surgeons (Chapter 4, p. 73).

The most common method for controlling airborne microbes is the plenum or turbulent ventilation system. Filtered air is introduced through vents high on the walls or in the ceiling of an OR. This mixes with the air already there. A slight positive pressure is maintained, and the mixture is discharged through vents placed low down at the maximum possible distance from the inlet. As the new air enters, it mixes with the old and the bacteria present are first diluted and then swept away. The incoming air is filtered to remove bacteria from it. In fact, most outside air contains remarkably few bacteria, nearly always many fewer, for instance, than are found inside an OR while it is in use. However, when tested years ago, fresh air was found to contain spores of *Clostridium tetani*, and so filtration became standard practice. It would be interesting to know if this is still necessary now that horses have disappeared from the streets of most cities. Sometimes, the bacterially contaminated air discharged from an OR is recycled to conserve the energy used to heat or cool it. If this is done (and some authorities advise against the practice because of the anaesthetic gases), then, of course, the air must be filtered before it is reused.

Clean-room technology, introduced to keep dust out of miniaturized electronic components during assembly, has had a major impact on OR ventilation. Because all airborne particles tend to be confused with microbes (Chapter 2, p. 30) filtration has been elaborated and particles smaller than necessary are removed. This has a cost consequence. It is worth noting that there is no evidence that filtration of the air supplied to ORs to the standards necessary in electronic clean rooms prevents surgical sepsis. Although microbes are very small, they almost always ride on rafts that are much larger than themselves.

The more air blown through a room, the greater the dilution of bacteria and the lower the bacterial count achieved. At some point, a balance is struck between the rates at which bacteria are added to the air by the occupants, and that at which they are removed by ventilation. The flow of air can be measured in 'air changes per hour', calculated by dividing the total volume of air delivered each hour by the volume of the OR. The maximum number of changes possible is determined by the noise and draught created, and the capital and revenue costs of the machinery.

Some years ago 16 changes an hour were thought adequate, now 20 or more are called for. The maximum possible may be about 30. Formerly, bacteriological standards were set for ORs, based on the maximum allowable number of bacteria-carrying particles in a cubic foot or cubic meter ($=35.3 \, \text{ft}^3$) of air. Although these numeric standards have been abandoned in favour of the physical criteria just given, they are still of interest and may even be of use in places where details of airflows are unknown. They ranged between 10 and 175 per m^3 ($<1-5 \, \text{per ft}^3$), depending on the country of origin and type of surgery. Neurosurgery and orthopaedic surgery were the most demanding. The counts quoted were the maximum acceptable during periods of quiet operating. Counts always rise markedly at the beginning and end of surgery, when levels of physical activity are high. In an OR that has been empty for an hour or so, the count should be zero.

For those without the slit sampler or other device required to make direct counts of airborne bacteria, settle plates may be used. A 90 mm (3.5 in) Petri dish of blood or nutrient agar is exposed at some convenient place near the operating table for an hour. After incubation overnight, the number of colonies that develop are counted, and identified, if required. To convert the number of colonies that develop after incubation into an approximation of the number of bacteria-carrying particles per m^3, the count is divided by 0.13, or by 4.5 for ft^3 (Williams *et al.*, 1966).

It is often suggested that an OR should be 'rested' to allow the bacterial count to return to a low level when an operation has been completed, particularly after a 'dirty' case. The time taken for the airborne count to fall to one-twentieth of its former level is three minutes at 20 changes an hour, or just under four at 16. As the entry of the next patient will put the count up again to the original level, anything more than a break of a few minutes has no microbiological logic. A rest may be thought necessary because pathogenic bacteria have escaped from an infected patient or his or her wound. The release of a significant number of pathogens into the air is unlikely. In the case of the skin, this is because the patient is immobile, and from a wound because any bacteria there are trapped in sticky liquid. Most 'dirty' cases are nothing of the kind. In this connection, a smell may be thought to indicate airborne contamination by microbes. In fact, smells indicate the presence of chemicals, not bacteria, in the air. Bacteria may produce smelly chemicals, but to do this they must be actively growing in a nutrient environment. They cannot do it when they are suspended in the air.

In any case, theatre staff carry most of the important pathogens among their own normal flora. Up to 50% of the population carry *Staph. aureus* and 100% carry *Cl. perfringens*. Both organisms, the latter the most important cause of gas gangrene, can be found in small numbers in the air of ORs much of the time. These have come from the bodies of the OR staff, and so again microbiology does not support the need for a rest. Part of the 'resting' period may be used to mop out the theatre. In the absence of soiling by body fluids, this has no useful purpose. In fact, it keeps the airborne count high due to the physical exertion of the cleaner. Routine cleaning on a daily basis is all that is necessary. Disinfectants add nothing useful to the process.

Another way of bringing air into an OR is by the laminar flow method. This introduces air from a part of the ceiling immediately over the operating table or from a wall close to it, so that the area round the patient and scrubbed operating team are enveloped in a steady downward or horizontal flow of filtered air. This produces the ultra-clean condition mentioned in Chapter 4 (p. 73), and is very effective as a way of washing away bacteria released from the skin of the operating team. However, the need for expensive high-efficiency particulate air (HEPA) filtration of the incoming air has not been explained.

The instruments and other surgical necessities exposed during an operation have an area many times greater than the average wound. Airborne microbes are more likely to get into a wound because they have fallen on to an instrument than by falling directly into the wound itself. Instruments should be exposed to the air for as short a time as possible. In some ODs, trolleys required for an operation are prepared during the preceding one. This is not recommended, though if it is to be done the instruments should be laid out in conditions no less good than they will meet when they are eventually used.

Of course, ODs are not driven by microbiological considerations alone. The difficulty is that practices that may be desirable for other reasons may for convenience (or out of ignorance) be supported by spurious microbiological ideas. If the real reason for wanting to rest an OR is that it is some of the staff who need the rest and a cup of coffee as well, it does not help to invent a microbiological fairy tale to justify it. Over the years, those who hear such tales come to believe them. This may be one of the reasons why individual microbiological fantasies have taken root and grown to become part of the self-perpetuating web of mystery common in operating departments.

INTENSIVE CARE UNITS

It is generally agreed that ICUs are hotbeds of HAI. This is illustrated in Table 6.1, where use is made of more of the data collected during the study in NUH Singapore mentioned in Chapter 2, p. 17 and p. 19. From this Figure it is clear that the chance of acquiring an infection in the three major adult ICUs in NUH was 3.5 times higher than in the rest of the hospital, and that in these units 100 infected patients would suffer 144 infections with 160 imputed pathogens. In the neonatal ICU the comparable figures are 3.4, 122 and 139. Outside ICUs 100 infected patients suffered from 115 infections with 123 pathogens. Compared with the risk in places where infections were least frequent ('other departments', Figure 2.2) patients in these ICUs were 18 times more likely to suffer at least one attack of HAI. The reason why a patient with one HAI is more likely to acquire a second is discussed in Chapter 2 (p. 18).

It is not difficult to find the cause of the high incidence of HAI in ICUs. Patients admitted to these units are selected precisely because they are seriously ill, and so are certain to be suffering from at least some immunocompromise from the outset. Their immune competence is reduced further as various life-support systems are attached to them. One or more intravascular lines, an endotracheal tube and a urinary catheter are commonplace. Each of these devices is associated with a significant added risk of infection (Chapter 5, p. 91). Patients in ICUs are handled by staff with greater frequency, and are more likely to be prescribed antimicrobial drugs than patients elsewhere. This explains why second and third infections (as well as primary ones) are more

Table 6.1 The pathogens causing HAI and the rates of infection detected in adult and neonatal ICUs in NUH Singapore (Chapter 2, p. 19), compared with those in the rest of the hospital

Pathogens	% HAI due to named pathogens in:		
	ICUs Adult*	Neonatal	Rest of Hospital
Escherichia coli	6	5	14
Klebsiella spp.	14	6	16
Enterobacter spp.	3	3	2
Proteus spp.	2	1	5
P. aeruginosa	14	3	8
Acinetobacter spp.	9	2	4
All Gram-negative rods	48	20	49
ORSA	6	15	12
MARSA	17	32	11
Staph. epidermidis	1	15	2
Candida spp.	13	2	4
Others	15	16	22
Infecting pathogens/1000 patients	144	124	32
Infections/1000 patients	130	109	30
Infected patients/1000	90	89	26

* Adult medical, surgical and cardiothoracic ICUs.
Key: ORSA, 'ordinary' *Staph. aureus*; MARSA, methicillin and aminoglycoside resistant *S. aureus*.

common here than in other parts of the hospital, and why these infections are more often polymicrobic.

The management of patients in ICUs is complex, requiring many special medical and nursing skills, and much complicated and expensive equipment. This is why patients who need these resources are concentrated in special units where they get the best available treatment applied in the most cost-effective way. As always, such benefits carry a penalty. Severely immunocompromised patients are much more susceptible to infection. When concentrated into ICUs, they are cared for by highly trained staff, drawn from among a small pool of individuals. The staff are regularly exposed to the special hospital strains of microbes generated in ICUs, and so they are more likely to become temporary or permanent carriers of them. Antimicrobials are prescribed with great frequency, and are often chosen from a very short list. All this ensures that infections, when they occur, are with similar multi-resistant bacteria. The result is that debilitated patients are infected frequently and severely with organisms often of low pathogenicity that are more difficult and expensive to treat. Infections are the major contributor to the heavy morbidity and mortality experienced by patients in ICUs. Because the organisms responsible are not a serious threat to healthy people, staff are not at risk of disease by being exposed to them, even when they become a carrier.

The distribution of HAI and of the pathogens that caused it in the ICUs in NUH (Chapter 2, p. 19 and p. 27) are compared with those in the rest of the hospital in Table 6.1. The main difference between the pathogens that caused HAI in these places is that in ICUs the generally more sensitive bacteria like *E. coli* and 'ordinary' *Staph. aureus* were replaced by more resistant organisms. The replacements in NUH differ from those described in some earlier reports. This may be due to growing use made in the 1980s of the expanding range of third-generation cephalosporins. These seem to encourage the emergence of methicillin- (and, of course, cephalosporin-) resistant *Staph. aureus* as a major hospital pathogen. As expected, this organism in both its methicillin sensitive and resistant forms are the predominant pathogens in the neonatal ICU.

In the face of the problems enumerated, the total prevention of infection in ICUs is a forlorn hope. The best that can be achieved is to reduce their number to some as yet undefined minimum. Many of them are self-infections of the autogenous sort, and some are cross-infections (Chapter 2, p. 28). Other than in burns units (Chapter 6, p. 140), environmental infections are only important if there is an accident or major carelessness. These usually involve the wet environment, particularly apparatus that contains liquid or collects condensation (Chapters 5, p. 91 and 6, p. 141). This generalization breaks down in the case of some transplant patients who are unusually susceptible to fungal infections, particularly with *Aspergillus* spp., the spores of which are transmitted through the air.

Other than as just noted, there is little evidence that the dry environment or the air contribute significantly to the rate of infection in ICUs; indeed, the opposite is the case (Bauer *et al.*, 1990). For this reason, expensive ventilation systems are only called for in special circumstances (in some transplant units, for example), and such things as overshoes, special headgear or adhesive mats at the entrance are not required. Masks (Chapter 5, p. 102) and gowns (Haque and Chagla, 1989) contribute little or nothing to the control of infection, and special disinfection is not necessary. The part played by clothing worn by staff in the transfer of infection is difficult to assess (Chapter 5, p. 101). This probably means that it is not very important, though it may play a small part. To reduce the risk and to protect clothing from direct contact with heavily contaminated sites or splashes, plastic aprons may be used when performing such procedures as endotracheal suction. These provide more protection than fabric gowns, though if satisfactory gowns made of waterproofed or other impervious material are available they would be preferable. This is probably more important if the task in hand involves a risk of significant contamination of arms or shoulders left unprotected by the usual plastic aprons. These areas may come into direct contact with patients more often in neonatal and burns units.

In ICUs as everywhere, the hands of staff are the main culprit responsible for the transfer of bacteria that colonize or infect patients (Chapter 5, p. 89). Hands commonly acquire bacterial pathogens as temporary residents by contact with patients who are already colonized or infected. Less often, but with disproportionately major significance, a bacterial pathogen can become part of the resident flora of the hands of a member of staff (Chapter 2, p. 31 and 5, p. 89). In either case, hospital bacteria are transferred with great efficiency to colonize and then infect a new patient. This route would be broken if each patient could be tended by staff on an individual basis. Although this may be attempted by providing a nurse for each patient, the attempt breaks down because it cannot be done for doctors, physiotherapists, respiratory and X-ray technicians, venipuncturists and the like. Even for nurses, the arrangement usually fails at night. Of course, the situation is much worse if ICUs are crowded or understaffed, or if they are provided with inadequate handwashing facilities.

In practice, the methods that ought to be used to prevent HAI in ICUs are exactly the same as those that should be used everywhere. The difference lies in the exceptional sensitivity to infection of the patients concerned, compounded by the intensity of their exposure to the risk of it. The result is that small breaks in technique that might not cause harm elsewhere are not forgiven in ICUs. The documented failure of staff to wash their hands (Chapter 5, p. 89) means that little will be gained by looking elsewhere for the cause of infections in ICUs, though the expensive pursuit of imaginary problems can easily develop into a cult, as it has in operating departments (above, p. 131). Though it could have a dramatic effect, simply to impose proper hand hygiene (if this were possible) is not the whole answer. Washing hands properly at the proper frequency would consume so much time as to affect staffing levels. It is also probable that sore hands would result, arguably producing an even greater problem with infection (Chapter 5, p. 90). This is an area that calls for new thinking.

Overall, a balance should be struck between the good and the harm done in ICUs. Some conclusion might be reached if this were

attempted at the level of patient survival, though not without difficulty. If the question of cost were then added, the difficulty would
intensify. Because health care is rationed everywhere, it would be
necessary to examine the justification for the high cost of ICUs, where
despite best efforts mortality may exceed 25%. The money spent on
each patient in an ICU would pay for the treatment of several in an
ordinary ward, who would have a much better chance of survival and
be more likely to return to a full, active life. Arguments over this issue
lie more in the moral and political arenas than in the medical one. It is
as well that the average doctor or nurse is not required to make the
choice.

BURNS UNITS

A burn wound is unusually susceptible to infection for two reasons.
First, a burn provides an area where water and nutrients are plentiful,
ideal for bacterial growth. Secondly, in a burn the normal defences
against bacterial invasion are weakened or absent. Not only is the
protective epidermis removed, but the initial coagulum and later a
slough prevent phagocytic cells, antibodies and the like from reaching
the area where bacterial multiplication can take place. Colonization of
the surface of a burn is therefore inevitable, even involving organisms
that have lost their power to infect normal tissue due to drying of their
surfaces (Chapters 2, p. 35 and 4, p. 65). In addition, a burn is a
powerful immunosuppressive agent, and so the body may be unable to
react to prevent colonization from becoming an infection. Although it
is difficult to determine clinically the point at which this change takes
place, its eventual effect is all too obvious. Patients with extensive
burns who survive the initial injury suffer a significant mortality later,
mostly as a result of infection.

Lives are saved by aggressive resuscitation immediately following a
burn. Proper care will prevent the injury from extending unnecessarily,
and in the end skin grafting is often required. The skills that contribute
to this process are best applied in burns units, which are specialist
ICUs that keep their patients longer than usual. As practically everything said about ICUs above (p. 136) applies to burns units, that
section should be read together with this one.

However, there are differences between an ordinary ICU and a
burns unit, and as these tend to make the control of infection more
difficult, they are important. Burns wounds whether colonized or
infected are uniquely prolific sources of bacteria. The sheer weight of
numbers makes routes for the transmission of infection that are of little

or no importance elsewhere become significant in a burns unit (Ransjo and Hambraeus, 1982). Of course, hands are still the principal route of transmission, but clothing, the environment and the air all play a part. The prolonged treatment of burns patients ensures that all the routes along which microbes can spread remain open for a long time. Even if transmission by hands could be controlled, infections would still be a problem in burns units. Conversely, because burns units are so different, the techniques used to control infection in them should not be applied uncritically to other areas. This has happened in the past, with expensive consequences (Colebrook, 1948).

The bacteria that cause infections in a given burns unit at any one time tend to be indistinguishable. The causes of this phenomenon were described for ICUs, but for the reasons just given, they apply to burns units with greater force. *Staph. aureus* (including MARSA) and a variety of Gram-negative organisms, chiefly *P. aeruginosa*, are the most common pathogens. Formerly, the more pathogenic *Strep. pyogenes* was also common, but it is now unusual. Each unit seems to provide a special niche that favours one or other of the major pathogens or, perhaps, a group of them which come and go over periods of months or years. The conditions in different units that favour one pathogen over another have not been defined, though they deserve study.

It is generally agreed that infection is inevitable with burns involving more than about 30% of the body surface. In these cases, control depends on the judicious use of antimicrobials. Otherwise, the precautions decribed for ICUs apply, noting the importance of the arms as well as the hands of staff in transmission (Burnett and Norman, 1990). To these may be added filtered ventilation and special clothing. A burns unit sited in a general hospital is an important permanent reservoir of pathogens that may spread to other patients. The physical segregation of burns units should be as complete as possible, and the staff working in them should not be transferred thoughtlessly to other areas, particularly to ICUs or oncology units.

WET ENVIRONMENTS

Life is impossible without water. Most living things die rapidly if deprived of it, though some can 'hibernate', if necessary for years, until water returns. In the absence of water, microbes cease to multiply, and most begin to die more or less quickly. Some last longer than others, but excepting the bacteria that form spores, only a few survive longer than a period measured in minutes or hours unless they are protected from lethal desiccation by, for instance, being embedded in material containing protein.

Microbes can cause an infection only if they are present in significant numbers, and can reach a victim. A totally dry environment that is also clean is remarkably safe, and it becomes safer as time passes, so long as new microbes are not added. A wet environment is the exact opposite. Unless special precautions are taken, it may be microbially dangerous at the beginning and it is likely to become increasingly so with time. Despite this, a wet environment is only a potential hazard if there is a vector or vehicle to convey any microbes it contains to a portal of entry where they can initiate an infection (Chapter 2, p. 28). On this basis, things that are wet can be identified immediately as being potentially dangerous, and they can be distinguished very clearly from dry items that are unlikely to be a problem. Wet environments in hospitals include intravenous and other liquid medications, dialysis, irrigation and rinsing fluids, medical equipment that contains liquids or collects it in the form of condensation, disinfecting and antiseptic solutions, food and drink, all plumbing, wet cleaning equipment, waste and sewerage systems, and parts of air-conditioning plants and hydrotherapy pools. To make the list complete, wet linen, wet bedpans, urinals and bowls, surfaces left wet after cleaning and ornamental water and flower vases must be added. However, unless a patient drinks the water from a flower vase, or it is used to irrigate a wound, the latter is only a reservoir and not a real source of infection (Chapter 2, p. 28).

Although there are wide variations, bacteria or fungi of one kind or another can multiply in most of the fluids found in hospitals, from distilled water to dilute solutions of disinfectants. The more pathogenic bacteria generally grow poorly or even fail to survive in many liquids. On the other hand, weak pathogens or free-living bacteria that are normally non-pathogenic may multiply to reach very large populations. Such liquid is inherently poisonous, even if the microbes cannot multiply in tissue to cause an infection. Fluids in this state are normally kept at bay by intact body surfaces, but medical procedures open routes that may allow them to reach privileged surfaces and internal tissues. Of course, debilitated hospital patients are specially vulnerable to an insult of this kind.

The only fluids that can be guaranteed as being microbiologically safe are those that have been prepared with great care to exclude microbes at every stage of manufacture, and have been sterilized properly (usually in an autoclave) inside a hermetically sealed final container that is still intact. Once the container has been damaged or opened, the fluid is compromised, and the chances that it will remain sterile diminish progressively as time passes. The importance of this varies with the purpose to which the fluid is to be put. An intravenous infusion, for example, requires more elaborate care than a can of soft drink, but the principles are the same. As is the case with food, refrigeration slows down, and freezing halts the multiplication of bacteria and fungi.

Modern plumbing and the wet parts of air-conditioning systems are happy hunting grounds for whole armies of mostly non- or weakly pathogenic microbes. It should be remembered that even high-quality drinking water is not sterile, and hot water may not be hot enough for long enough to disinfect itself. Depending on the plumbing system, hospital water may contain large numbers of bacteria. These usually pose no threat to healthy members of staff, but may be dangerous to patients. They may include *Legionella pneumophila*, the cause of legionellosis. The air delivery ducts of air-conditioning systems are (or should be) dry, so air does not pick up microbes as it passes through them, but this may not be true where there is water in the system. Where air-conditioning systems, air-cooling plants and humidifiers are wet inside, they are suspect. The dangers can be reduced by good design and regular skilled maintenance.

The wet environment is controlled by limiting its extent as far as possible, and by applying sensible controls to what is left. These include the keeping of sterile fluids intended for parenteral use sealed in their containers until the last possible moment, taking great care when making additions of medications to infusions, and limiting the time any delivery system is kept attached to a patient. Nasogastric feeds used for enteral hyperalimentation have been identified as an important source of HAI (Thurn *et al.*, 1990). These feeds should be prepared in scrupulously clean and disinfected equipment. They should be kept refrigerated until needed, and should not be stored for more than a few hours. Remember that while fluids are being run into patients, they are exposed to room temperature. If they are con-taminated, bacterial multiplication will continue at a compound rate for however long the process takes.

There is no place for regular, routine microbiological testing of the environment, wet or dry, with the possible exception of infant feeds if these are prepared in the hospital, or piped water if the quality of the supply is uncertain or variable. Microbiological testing is required when a problem arises, and it should be directed at its most probable cause. Testing should cease when a solution has been found, applied and been shown to work. When what might be a source of microbes causing infections has been identified, remember that this may in fact be just another victim of the real source, yet to be discovered.

FURTHER READING

Ayliffe, G. A. J. and Lawrence, T. C. (eds) (1985) Symposium on infection control in burns. *J. Hosp. Infect.*, **6** (Supplement B), 1–66.

REFERENCES

Bauer, T. M., Ofner, E., Just, H. M. *et al.* (1990) An epidemiological study assessing the relative importance of airborne and direct contact transmission of microorganisms in a medical intensive care unit. *J. Hosp. Infect.*, **15**, 301–9.

Bethune, D. W., Blowers, R., Parker, M. *et al.* (1965) Dispersal of *Staphylococcus aureus* by patients and surgical staff. *Lancet*, **i**, 480–3.

Burnett, I. A. and Norman, P. (1990) *Streptococcus pyogenes*: an outbreak on a burns unit. *J. Hosp. Infect.*, **15**, 173–6.

Colebrook, L. (1948) The control of infection in burns. *Lancet*, **i**, 893–9.

Dankert, J., Zijlstra, J. B. and Lubberding, H. (1979) A garment for use in the operating theatre: the effect upon bacterial shedding. *J. Hyg., Camb.*, **82**, 7–14.

Haque, K. N. and Chagla, A. H. (1989) Do gowns prevent infection in neonatal intensive care units? *J. Hosp. Infect.*, **14**, 159–62.

Laufman, H., Montefusco, C., Siegal, J. D. *et al.* (1980) Scanning electron microscopy of moist bacterial strike-through of surgical materials. *Surg. Gynae. Obstet.*, **150**, 165–70.

Lewis, D. A., Weymont, G., Nokes, C. M. *et al.* (1990) A bacteriological study of the effect on the environment of using a one- or two-trolley system in theatre. *J. Hosp. Infect.*, **15**, 35–53.

May, K. R. and Pomeroy, N. P. (1973) Bacterial dispersion from the body surface, in *Airborne Transmission and Airborne Infection*, (eds J. F. Ph. Hers and K. C. Winkler) Oosthoek, Utrecht, pp. 426–34.

Meers, P. D. and Yeo, G. A. (1978) Shedding of bacteria and skin squames after handwashing. *J. Hyg., Camb.*, **81**, 99–105.

Ransjo, U. and Hambraeus, A. (1982) When to wash walls in ward rooms? *J. Hosp. Infect.*, **3**, 81–6.

Spiers, R., Bernard, H., O'Grady, F. *et al.* (1965) Increased dispersal of skin bacteria into the air after shower-baths. *Lancet*, **i**, 478–80.

Thurn, J., Crossley, K., Gerdts, A. *et al.* (1990) Enteral hyperalimentation as a source of nosocomial infection. *J. Hosp. Infect.*, **15**, 203–17.

Williams, R. E. O., Blowers, R., Garrod, L. P. *et al.* (1966) *Hospital Infection, Causes and Prevention*, 2nd edn, Lloyd-Luke, London, p. 372.

Chapter 7

Service Departments

OCCUPATIONAL HEALTH, STAFF VACCINATION AND SAFETY

Even when it is not a legal obligation, employers should make a point of caring for the health and well-being of their employees. Many hospitals operate a comprehensive staff health programme, providing medical examination on entry, immunization, and a 'walk-in' service for medical problems (including injuries) that arise at work. Such an occupational health service will monitor infections that might affect employability either temporarily or permanently. It should also supervise the management of HCWs who have suffered an accident that exposes them to the risk of infection, particularly with the hepatitis B and human immunodeficiency viruses. The service should include counselling. ICTs should maintain close links with such organizations, and ICCs ought to produce guidelines for the immunization of HCWs. In some hospitals, arrangements for the care of staff are less complete, and in others they are rudimentary or totally lacking.

Apart from any legal or moral responsibility for employees as part of effective management, the duty of care in respect of infection is far stronger in hospitals. An HCW with open tuberculosis may infect dozens of patients, or one with mild chickenpox or shingles may be the source of a lethal infection in a child being treated for leukaemia. On the other hand, a HCW may contract hepatitis B or HIV infection from a patient, or a pregnant HCW may lose her fetus because of rubella. Management should seek to prevent these kinds of accidents by setting up and supporting the kind of organization outlined above.

A vital part of the programme is staff education. Induction courses for different groups of HCWs on first employment should include instruction on how to avoid infecting themselves or the patients they serve. The importance of reporting all accidents should be stressed. Insistence on a 'safety first' attitude to work is part of the process. This will range from the right way to lift objects so as to avoid back injuries, to the proper handling of sharp instruments to avoid infections.

These messages should continually be reinforced by in-service education.

Integral to a staff health programme is an immunization policy. This should be designed to protect HCWs from infections they might contract from patients, and to protect patients from infections they might acquire from HCWs. Requirements will vary according to the health problems in the community served by the hospital, and according to the categories of staff. A review would include tuberculosis (which would require a decision on the need for chest X-rays of staff), rubella, poliomyelitis, diphtheria, tetanus and hepatitis B. In the case of varicella, the supposed or actual immune status of HCWs might be recorded, to aid with staff allocation to high-risk areas.

CENTRAL STERILE SUPPLY

Lister's introduction of antiseptic surgery was a singular event, dated precisely to 1867. By contrast, the replacement of the antiseptic method by the unfortunately named aseptic surgery (Chapter 6, p. 131) seems to have begun independently in several countries at slightly different times. The technique continued to develop for many years – indeed, in some respects it is still incomplete. However, right from the beginning one major requirement separated aseptic from antiseptic surgery. This followed from the need to sterilize surgical paraphernalia. The first completely effective method to be adopted is still in use today. The steam sterilizer or autoclave was originally adapted for medical use in Germany in 1886.

What happened next differed in various parts of the world. In many places, boiling water was used to make metal surgical equipment safe, while fabrics – gowns, drapes, dressings and so on – were autoclaved. These practices spread from operating departments into wards and clinics, where the separate use of so-called boiling sterilizers for metal items and of autoclaves for dressings continued. Each ward and clinic would have its own boiler, looked after by nurses. The large, more complicated autoclaves were kept out of sight. The early machines with their masses of exposed pipes, valves and dials were given to making loud noises and to violent discharges of quantities of hot water and steam. It was difficult to find sufficient knowledgeable people to take responsibility for these rather fearsome objects, and the duty often fell to junior persons with strong nerves and limited imagination. In these circumstances, autoclaves were often badly misused.

These arrangements were clearly unsatisfactory. Sterilization to modern standards was not often achieved, and some equipment was dangerous to users. Due to the massive over-kill inherent in an autoclave (Chapter 5, p. 109) not many accidents were recorded that were the result of a failure of sterilization. More notable was the inadequacy of management and the lack of supervision. To these deficiencies was added the low cost-effectiveness of using ward nurses to prepare one by one each of the settings needed for the enormous number of procedures carried out every day. What was required was a central service to perform the whole function, to produce and distribute standard, securely wrapped sterile packs each containing what was necessary for a given process. This was recognized and acted upon in the USA in the 1930s. In the 1940s, the idea and the practice spread widely, partly as a result of military need.

The development of central services created a demand for a whole new range of machinery. This comprised more efficient high- and low-temperature autoclaves, gas sterilizers, sophisticated apparatus for washing and cleaning instruments, and other appliances. The appearance of ever more complex and expensive diagnostic and therapeutic equipment added a new dimension. Many of these items are made of modern materials that cannot be resterilized by traditional means. This added to existing problems the need to invent and monitor new methods and apparatus for treating them so as to ensure that, at least, they are acceptably disinfected (Chapter 5, p. 106 and p. 122).

With these developments, a new increasingly sophisticated industry appeared in hospitals. The need for novel technical and managerial skills led to the development of special training programmes and the appearance of new paramedical specialists. Depending on circumstances, a variety of patterns (and nomenclatures) emerged. In some places, a single central sterile supply department (CSSD) grew up to cater for the needs of wards, clinics, operating departments and, sometimes, for medical services in the community as well. In others, separate services were provided, most often in the form of CSSDs plus theatre sterile supply units (TSSUs) that were often sited within operating departments. As more items appeared that had to be disinfected, CSSDs were sometimes renamed hospital sterilization and disinfection units (HSDUs).

The procedures carried out in a central sterilizing unit can be broken down into reception of used equipment, which is then washed, dried, inspected, and repacked together with whatever disposable items are required. Packs are then sterilized and stored (sometimes within a use-by period) until they are needed. These procedures are modified as necessary to accommodate special items, or equipment that can only withstand disinfection. In some places, parts or the whole of the unit performing these functions are required to conform to 'clean room' conditions, with staff wearing lint-free clothing and working in HEPA filtered air. This is another example of extreme and expensive measures being introduced intuitively, without proof of need.

Difficulties may arise when equipment returned to the central unit has been used on a patient who is 'infectious'. Sometimes there is concern that staff in the unit might be infected by handling the items during the early parts of the recycling process. What some people regard as 'infectious' in fact may not be hazardous for staff at all. A good example of an imaginary problem is MARSA, but concern about hepatitis B and to a lesser extent HIV infection cannot be dismissed so easily. Some centres require that equipment used in such cases is returned either having been exposed to some disinfectant or actually immersed in one. The idea that this makes for greater safety ignores the fact that many patients with these infections pass through hospitals without being identified. Equipment used for a variety of invasive procedures on such patients is returned to the central unit and reprocessed without special precautions. Although there is no record of a worker in a central unit having been infected in this way, the concern is genuine and cannot be ignored.

Rather than the use of chemical disinfectants, which is expensive, messy and ecologically unfriendly, it should be possible to pass all instruments through a mechanical washer-disinfector immediately on receipt in the central unit, before they are touched at all. This extension of universal precautions (Chapter 5, p. 94) means that no special segregation is needed for 'infectious' items. The preliminary process makes everything safe to handle, provided elementary care is taken. If this is done, there is no need for any instruments to be cleaned or decontaminated before reaching the CSSD. More expensive washer-sterilizers are not necessary for this purpose. They have a reputation for baking blood on to instruments rather than removing it.

A washer-disinfector is an extremely useful piece of machinery (Anon, 1983). It appears in hospitals in many guises. The technology is well established as it is the same as that found in a domestic dishwasher. It operates on a principle similar to that used in laundries (below, p. 152) in that a cold rinse is followed by a hot wash, probably with a detergent, and the process ends with a hot rinse at about 80°C for between one and two minutes. This final temperature varies, and so does the time, and figures of 65°C for 10 minutes to 90°C for a few seconds have been quoted. The point is that provided the washing cycle is really efficient, the pasteurizing final rinse has little left to do except make the object being treated so hot that it conveniently dries itself on exposure to colder air. Machines employing this general principle are used in wards for cleaning and disinfecting bedpans and urinals, elsewhere for processing plastic or rubber anaesthetic equipment, in kitchens for cleaning and disinfecting eating utensils and in CSSDs as just indicated.

Of course, when purchasing equipment of this sort, the claims of manufacturers should not be accepted at face value, and machines should be checked both for their washing efficiency and the time and temperature achieved in the rinse cycle. Once installed, they need to be checked regularly for mechanical function, and the temperature they reach. For this purpose, cheap, easily portable electronic thermometers are available. These instruments are attached by fine wires to small probes that can be inserted into the chamber of machines while they are operating. Some models are equipped with a variety of probes for different applications, including the measurement of airflows. Slightly more sophisticated models include a recorder so that a permanent record may be made over a period of time. ICTs should be equipped with such apparatus.

KITCHENS

Those responsible for hospital catering face unique problems. They must try to produce and distribute a palatable, safe diet to people scattered through one or more large buildings, most of whom cannot assemble at central points, and some of whom have particular and perhaps complex dietary requirements. The service must be available 24 hours a day, 365 days a year, is often subject to budgetary restriction, and may be provided from inadequate, outdated kitchens. Many of the customers are patients, and so have been selected precisely because they are already sick. Sick people are more likely than the healthy to develop food-related illness, and to die of it. The margin for error is much reduced. This scene is set in a medical environment where the result of even minor mistakes are much more likely to be noticed, investigated and reported. Because there is usually a microbiology laboratory on the site, it is more probable that the cause will be damningly identified. It is not surprising that outbreaks of food poisoning seem to be more common in hospitals than elsewhere.

Understandable it may be, but not excusable. Microbial food poisoning is avoidable, and results from elementary mistakes in food hygiene. Most food poisoning in hospitals is of bacterial origin, and the organisms responsible (often salmonellas or *Cl. perfringens*) are nearly always present in small numbers in the food when it arrives at the hospital. The other main cause, *Staph. aureus* is usually added to the food in the kitchen, also in small numbers, by carriers of the bacterium who comprise up to 50% of the population, or by someone suffering from sepsis due to it. Salmonella infections in hospitals are discussed further in Chapter 4 (p. 85).

A surprisingly large proportion of the food offered for sale internationally contains small numbers of food-poisoning microbes. More of it is contaminated in the kitchen, as described. In either case, proper handling of the food can prevent this rather common contamination from becoming dangerous. The reason is that, as with all poisons, it is not so much the presence of the poison that matters, but rather how much there is of it. In the case of bacteria, it is necessary to have at least many hundreds or, more often, very many thousands in each gram of food before the toxic threshold is reached. Bacteria can multiply in most kinds of food, but only at certain temperatures. For nearly all the bacteria that matter, multiplication is most rapid between about 20°C and 40°C. Below freezing (food freezer temperature, nominally −20°C) multiplication stops altogether. Between 4°C and 8°C (efficient refrigerator temperatures), multiplication is so slow as to be effectively stopped in the short term (a few days). This is why **effective** refrigeration is such a vital part of food hygiene. An overloaded or inefficient refrigerator may be unable to achieve a safe temperature under any circumstances, and even if it does, anything hot put in it will take an unacceptably long time to chill. In either case, bacterial multiplication will continue for longer than it should.

Paradoxically refrigeration may encourage one foodborne pathogen that has recently come into prominence. *Listeria monocytogenes* continues to multiply slowly in the refrigerator (particularly when the temperature rises above 4°C or 5°C), so that food contaminated with it may in time come to contain an infectious dose of the bacterium. At the same time, effective chilling keeps the food 'wholesome' by preventing the growth of food-spoiling organisms. The listeria story is still unfolding as more and more mass-produced chilled food is distributed internationally. Because *L. monocytogenes* is an important pathogen for the immunocompromised, it may emerge as a problem in hospitals.

As the temperature of food rises to between 40°C and 50°C, bacterial multiplication ceases, and above 50°C heat begins to become lethal, though less so, of course, for the spores of *Cl. perfringens*. Thorough cooking is very destructive of bacteria, but it must be remembered that large joints of meat or poultry take longer to heat up. This is particularly true if they have been frozen and are not properly defrosted before cooking begins. Carefully processed food that is eaten immediately after adequate heating is very safe from a microbiological point of view.

It is unfortunate that thorough cooking makes some food unpalatable. Eating thus becomes a form of Russian roulette as some pathogenic microbes (and the enterotoxin of *Staph. aureus*) may escape destruction during a short exposure to heat.

Problems emerge if cooked food is stored prior to consumption. As the temperature of the food falls below about 40°C, any surviving bacteria start to multiply again. If the temperature stays in the 'danger zone' (10°C to 40°C) for long enough (an hour or two may suffice), the toxic threshold may be reached and those who consume the food will suffer from food poisoning. This can be avoided if heated food is kept hot (above 60°C) or if it is chilled **rapidly** to refrigerator temperature. This is a particular problem in hospitals because meals have to be distributed in relatively small amounts to many destinations. In these circumstances, it is difficult to keep food at the desired temperature. The answer lies in timing, discipline and efficient food trolleys. Of course, food that has to be reheated runs a double risk of being mishandled.

The rules are simple, and if they were obeyed food poisoning would be rare. They may be broken for a variety of reasons, including complaints about over-cooked food, pressure of work, inadequate facilities or the employment of poorly trained staff. Of course, food eaten raw or nearly so escapes the disinfecting effect of heat. Contamination of fruit and salads with gastrointestinal pathogens does not reach toxic levels if they have been properly handled and refrigerated. This does not always happen, and in many places these foods are at least suspect. Eggs may be contaminated with salmonellas, and so if eaten when they are inadequately cooked or raw can lead to food poisoning. Shellfish are always a gamble. Of course, salads and the like should be carefully washed and kept cold before being eaten.

Other points require attention. Separate refrigerators should be provided for fresh and cooked foods, to prevent the recontamination of a cooked item by contact with an uncooked one. All equipment and, in particular, slicers, mixers, blenders and other catering machinery, together with work surfaces, must be kept scrupulously clean, using an approved catering detergent or disinfectant with plenty of hot water. Grubby cloths should be banned, and machinery usually needs to be taken apart to clean it properly.

The general hygiene of the kitchen, and of the staff, must be considered. A clean kitchen is the hallmark of a staff who are professionally competent, and not under dangerous pressure. The importance of insects and other parasites has been discussed in Chapter 2 (p. 34). Staff suffering from diarrhoea or with septic skin lesions should not be allowed to work. Practice varies on the performance of routine laboratory examinations of the faeces of employees on first appointment, or subsequently. Although this should always be done to clear an employee for return to work after an attack of diarrhoea, the answer otherwise varies with the incidence of gastrointestinal infections in the community from which the employee comes. When this is low, routine examinations are not cost-effective, and an examination may be limited to the taking of a medical history and the ordering of cultures only in cases where there has been a recent stomach upset or a history of enteric fever at any time. When the incidence of gastrointestinal infections (and infestations) is high and, in particular, where typhoid or paratyphoid is common, faecal examinations ought to be done in every case, if the facilities exist.

One of the duties of the ICT is to visit and inspect hospital kitchens from time to time. If catering is done by a contractor, the ICC or ICT should be involved when tenders are invited to check that contracts are properly drawn up so far as hygiene is concerned.

LAUNDRY

Bedding, clothing, furnishings and the like make up the largest group of items used in hospitals today that have remained substantially untouched by the boom in disposables. It is a requirement that after use these should be treated by a process that renders them aesthetically acceptable, that is, clean and nicely presented for reuse, and safe (particularly microbiologically so), but does not unreasonably shorten their life. This is usually achieved by a process of washing in water followed by drying and pressing, that is, by laundering.

The laundry cycle consists of one or more cold or cool rinses, followed by washing at a raised temperature, further rinsing, water extraction, drying, pressing, folding and packing. Such things as detergents, bleaches, conditioners, starches and so on are added at various points. The whole process may be done by hand, or mechanized up to the level represented by a modern domestic washing machine, or beyond to the level possible using the sophisticated machinery available in large commercial laundries.

The initial cold or cool rinses wash off stains or other relatively soluble or loosely bound materials that have soiled fabrics. This is particularly important if any of them might otherwise be 'cooked' into the weave at a higher temperature. Natural egg white, for example, is easily washed out of a piece of cloth in cold water, but it is denatured and becomes insoluble in hot water and is then very difficult to remove. The same applies to blood and other protein-containing body fluids, and to a lesser extent to faeces. Washing at a raised temperature helps to extract less soluble materials, with assistance from detergents. The removal of dirt simultaneously removes microbes, which are also subjected to the disinfecting action of heat, and of any chemicals that are added. Further significant disinfection may be achieved in the drying and pressing parts of the cycle, depending on the temperature reached. High-quality cotton and linen fabrics withstand washing at temperatures up to the boiling point of water, though many modern materials used to make clothing would be destroyed at this temperature. In choosing the temperature used for washing, the amount of energy used should be considered. It has been calculated that high-temperature laundering accounts for perhaps 15% of a hospital's total energy requirement. The cost of this, together with the non-replaceable nature of most current energy sources, impose a need to use the lowest temperature that achieves the twin requirements of cleanliness and safety.

The hot part of the washing cycle may be performed at 71°C for a period of up to 30 minutes. Although vegetative bacteria and viruses (including HIV and almost certainly hepatitis B) are destroyed in less time, it is prolonged to ensure that all parts of the load in a commercial washer reach the required temperature. The final temperature used varies, but for hot cycles it has usually fallen between 65°C and 80°C. Washing at lower temperatures would seem to risk less complete disinfection, but direct experiment has shown that, provided products are treated by a modern process in modern machines and are clean when they emerge, they are likely to be substantially free of microbes (Blaser *et al.*, 1984; Tompkins *et al.*, 1988). Clean laundry does not need to be sterile other than in operating rooms or for sterile packs. In practice, if it is aesthetically acceptable, it is likely to be microbiologically safe.

Laundering is only a part of the continuous cycle through which fabrics pass until they are worn out. From the laundry, they should be returned to the linen store and issued to users in suitable containers to protect them from harm and keep them clean. What happens to them after use is more of a problem. Difficulties arise because some individuals perceive that soiled items being returned to the laundry are a hazard to people working there (compare CSSDs, above, p. 148). The dangers are greatly overestimated. At the hospital end, all that is required is to handle soiled items gently and pack them into impervious bags as quickly as possible. Gloves may be worn if they are obviously contaminated with body fluids or have been used by a patient in isolation in cases where hospital policy has judged this added precaution is necessary. Provided the bags are of reasonable quality, double-bagging is not required. The question then arises, do soiled items need to be categorized by the risks they pose to laundry workers?

This risk arises because laundries often prefer to sort soiled items prior to putting them into washers. This is to separate items requiring different forms of treatment, and to avoid expensive damage to machines due to metal items (forceps, bowls, scissors, etc.) that are not infrequently included in laundry bags by mistake. Although there are no reports of infections in operatives who perform this task, sorting items in this way carries a theoretical risk. Hospital laundry has been categorized as 'soiled' (used but not objectionably dirty or dangerous), 'foul' (soiled with blood or faeces, for instance) or 'infected' (an impossibility as it is not alive, but meaning **contaminated** with microbes **thought** to be hazardous). It may be foul and infected simultaneously. In most cases, so long as the person doing the sorting wears good quality gloves and a waterproof apron and boots and, perhaps, eye protection, has been trained to be careful and is provided with proper changing and handwashing or showering facilities, and can be trusted to follow instructions, there is almost no danger, even in theory.

However, the duty of care imposes a constraint, and it is difficult not to have a residual list of situations requiring greater precautions. These should not extend to infections such as those with MRSA, the hepatitis B virus or HIV, though emotion might overcome logic when laundry from cases of the latter is dealt with for the first time as a new problem. If smallpox still existed, this would certainly require extra precautions, as would some rare conditions like Lassa, Marburg or Ebola fevers, anthrax and plague. Laundry soiled with the faeces of patients with typhoid, dysentery and cholera might also be treated differently. In some hospitals, all linen that falls into the foul category is also dealt with differently. This can be justified if the people who sort the linen at their laundry cannot be trusted to apply the universal precautions (Chapter 5, p. 94) described in the last paragraph. These precautions are thought to be sufficient to protect hospital staff from the same hazard. Each hospital or group of related hospitals must decide how far to extend these special precautions, remembering that this has a cost consequence.

The special category of contaminated ('infected') linen, however defined, may be packed in bags made of plastic that dissolves in either cold or hot water, or that are stitched together with plastic thread that is soluble in this way. Laundry contained in these is put directly into washing machines without prior opening or sorting. It is then released into the water when the bag (or its stitching) dissolves. Depending on the type employed, this happens either in the cold or the hot part of the cycle.

Cold-water soluble bags or bags with cold-water soluble stitching have the problem that if items are wet when they are placed in them or if the bags are exposed to water (rain, for instance) when they are full, they may disintegrate, releasing their contents in inappropriate places. This is unacceptable. Hot-water soluble bags overcome this problem in part, but when using them it is sensible to wrap wet linen inside dry items. The temperature at which these bags dissolve seems to depend to some extent on the length of time they are exposed to water at any temperature. Their contents may still escape unexpectedly, particularly in warm and humid climates.

Even when they work perfectly, these bags suffer the disadvantage that their contents are not rinsed during the cold or cool part of the laundering cycle. There is then a risk that any foul laundry will be stained indelibly if, for instance, blood is cooked into fabrics when bags release their contents directly into hot water. Provided the amount of laundry categorized as infected is small, this risk may be accepted, but good laundry policies and strict discipline in their application are required if the volume is to be kept under control. The main requirement is to reduce to a minimum the number of infections for which soluble laundry bags are used. Hot-water soluble bags are not cheap, and so bags made of less expensive materials but stitched together with hot-water soluble thread might seem attractive. Unfortunately, the insoluble plastic of which the rest of the bag is made goes through the laundering process and may cause malfunctions if it gets caught in moving parts, or it may soften and melt in the drying or pressing phases of the cycle.

An alternative to the use of soluble bags is to pack linen requiring special treatment in distinctive bags made of waterproof material. The contents of these are emptied into a washing machine without any preliminary sorting. An old solution to the problem of foul linen was to sluice it in the ward before it was bagged. More recently, it was taken in specially identified bags to a central 'foul washer' situated in the hospital where it was rinsed in cold water prior to despatch to the laundry. Neither of t'.ese solutions is acceptable in modern conditions.

An important part of a laundry policy is to define and specify the types of laundry bag to be used. It is customary to have these made in certain easily distinguished colours, sometimes chosen on a regional or national basis. This is helpful when staff move between hospitals. Depending on the number of categories of laundry required, two, three or more types of bag are needed. A minimum is one each for soiled and infected items, plus a third bag for fabrics to be washed at lower temperatures if these are sorted at ward level. To avoid confusion, the colours must be chosen not to coincide with those used for bagging hospital waste (Chapter 5, p. 128).

DOMESTIC CLEANING

Hospitals should be bright and clean. A clean environment makes patients feel better and staff work more efficiently. Dirty hospitals (to be distinguished from old and shabby ones) used to be dangerous places. This was not so much because dirt caused disease, but because a dirty hospital, like a dirty kitchen, was a sure sign of a poorly trained, sloppy staff. Infections and dirt were both due to inadequate care. A cause-and-effect relationship between dirt and disease exists mainly in the minds of those who confuse the real causes of infection with aesthetic considerations.

The indirect relationship noted between dirt and disease held when people who cared for patients in a hospital were also responsible for its cleanliness. This is no longer always true. A separation of roles has sometimes been imposed to increase commercial competitiveness, or otherwise it has been the result of cost-cutting in centrally funded services. It is now possible to have a squeaky-clean hospital with low-grade clinical staff, poor diagnostic services and too much HAI, or a dirty hospital where dedicated and competent doctors and nurses work, backed up by good diagnostic departments, with a low incidence of HAI.

In most hospitals, the dry environment contributes very little as a cause of HAI (Chapter 2, p. 36). Of course, the psychological importance of cleanliness allows no compromise, but routine environmental disinfection adds nothing useful. Expensive and environmentally unfriendly chemical disinfectants are almost never needed. Other than where body fluids have been spilt, water and detergent is all that is required to clean floors, walls and other surfaces in all areas of the hospital, including operating rooms. The nature of the cleaning equipment does not matter from an infection control point of view. What does matter is that mops, squeegees and so on are washed clean after use, then dried and stored dry. Some people feel more comfortable if mop heads are autoclaved from time to time. There is no reason to think this is of any value. If mechanical floor scrubbers or, in particular, vacuum cleaners are used, any discharge of air from the machine should, on balance, be filtered. This is to avoid disseminating any of the more hardy pathogens that can be spread by the environmental airborne route (Chapter 2, p. 35).

Spills of body fluids are a potential hazard. However, even when the spill contains large numbers of microbial pathogens, the risk of infection to other patients or staff is low or very low, provided elementary precautions are taken. This is because microbes have to find a route or a vector if they are to reach a portal of entry to cause an infection. Microbes contained in more or less viscous body fluids cannot escape into the air without the application of a great deal of force. Gentle handling using appropriate apparatus while wearing cheap, non-sterile plastic gloves or even plastic bags on the hands makes the process safe. To increase the safety factor when the spill is semi-solid or a mixture of solids and liquid, any pathogens (at least those on the surface) may be disinfected before cleaning is attempted. Because the microbes that are most feared in this context are viruses, chlorine is often recommended for the purpose. This has been combined with absorbent granules in a commercial product that simultaneously disinfects and soaks up the liquids in a spill, making final cleaning easier. Otherwise, hypochlorite at the right concentration may be used (Chapter 5, p. 119). Remember, disinfectants do not act instantaneously. Do not start to clean up a spill until the disinfectant has acted for about 10 minutes. In the meantime, it can be covered with, for instance, absorbent paper towels. Final disposal is into the kind of plastic bag that is used for contaminated waste (Chapter 5, p. 124). With a liquid spill (of blood, for instance), the preliminary disinfection may be dispensed with if the material is allowed to soak into paper towels. In ORs, soiled drapes may be used, if they are absorbent. Whatever the approach, the area from which the spill has been removed is treated with fresh disinfectant before a final clean with detergent and water. If the place concerned is a confined one, adequate ventilation should be ensured.

'Terminal disinfection' was part of the routine in old fever hospitals. Unnecessary ritual still lingers in the procedures sometimes used when patients are discharged from isolation. Unless the room in which a patient with, say, typhoid has been nursed is visibly contaminated with fresh faeces (in which case the body fluids procedure just described is appropriate), nothing more than routine detergent-and-water cleaning is required. Walls do not need to be cleaned, unless they are dirty. Screens or curtains should not be laundered unless they are soiled. Bed linen that is not contaminated with faeces or urine needs no special treatment, provided the laundry is efficient (above, p. 152). Books and other items do not need to be fumigated. The same applies to other diseases, including most respiratory ones, substituting for faeces and urine the appropriate contaminated body fluid. Most pathogens do not survive well in a dry environment (Chapter 2, p. 23).

This is something of an oversimplification. The general impression that by wiping a surface all particulate matter is removed is supported by the commonplace observation that visible dust is readily swept away, particularly if a damp cloth or disposable wipe is used. In fact, this is not true of very small particles like bacteria, which adhere to surfaces much more firmly, and which may, in addition, lurk in the microscopic crevices or scratches that mark even a smooth object. For this reason, a significant number of the bacteria that were on a surface beforehand remain on it after it has been damp dusted. If a cloth that has remained damp for an hour or two after earlier use is employed rather than a disposable wipe, the action is likely to 'paint on' more bacteria than it removes. This is because bacteria, especially GNRs, have multiplied in the cloth in the interval. What happens next depends on how much water is left behind at the end of the process. If this is minimal, drying soon begins to kill the residual bacteria. If a surface is left wet, or if the damp dusting is repeated frequently (as may be the case in busy kitchens, above, p. 149) significant bacterial multiplication may take place in what has now become a wet environment (Chapter 6, p. 141). 'Clean and dry' is the watchword, and when this is adhered to, little harm will follow.

Cases of open tuberculosis (patients not yet treated in whom the site of a tuberculous infection communicates with the outside world) may be a little different. As noted in Chapter 2 (p. 35) tubercle bacilli have a remarkable ability to survive desiccation. In fact, careful washing with detergent and water will usually prevent their being resuspended in the air, which is the only place where they can do any harm. When cleaning is finished, the dirty water should be disposed of into a proper sewage system, and the wipe dealt with as clinical waste (Chapter 5, p. 124). However, with tuberculosis, the margin of safety is narrow, and there is a distant chance that bacteria left behind after wiping may survive for long enough eventually to be carried into the air. This becomes important when the number of tubercle bacilli is large, for example, where patients do not dispose of their sputum hygienically, where a proper sewage system does not exist and, in particular, where open pulmonary tuberculosis is common, perhaps due to AIDS. In these circumstances, a phenolic disinfectant at the concentration for dirty situations (Chapter 5, p. 120) may be applied before ordinary washing.

Domestic employees in hospitals are at only slightly greater risk of infection than members of the general community, other than as a result of needle-stick injuries (Chapter 5, p. 124). HCWs may have met a patient now in hospital with a diagnosis of tuberculosis, hepatitis B or HIV infection a day or two ago in a store, on an elevator or as the driver of a cab. The new factor is awareness, but a patient just admitted with an illness not yet diagnosed may be a greater danger. If proper care is taken, for instance, the application of universal precautions (Chapter 5, p. 94) the risk is very small. Personnel should be vaccinated against the most serious hazard, hepatitis B. Compared with employees in most other industries, HCWs work in a safe environment, but fear of infection is a powerful instinct. Alarm may be spread out of ignorance or be fomented deliberately as a ploy when negotiating for improved pay or conditions. Education is the answer, provided the educator is properly informed. Of course, there is no excuse for lack of care by management, and there is always room for improvement. It is as much a part of the duties of an ICT or an ICC to think about the health of staff as to be concerned for patients.

REFERENCES

Anon (1983) Disinfection in washing machines. *J. Hosp. Infect.*, **4**, 101–2.

Blaser, M. J., Smith, P. F., Cody, H. J. *et al.* (1984) Killing of fabric-associated bacteria in hospital laundry by low-temperature washing. *J. Infect. Dis.*, **149**, 48–57.

Tompkins, D. S., Johnson, P. and Fittall, B. R. (1988) Low-temperature washing of patients' clothing; effects of detergent with disinfectant and a tunnel drier on bacterial survival. *J. Hosp. Infect.*, **12**, 51–8.

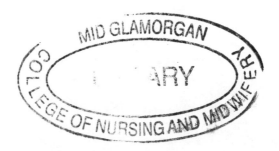

Chapter 8

Postscript

WHAT FUTURE FOR INFECTION CONTROL?

The prevention of infection in hospitals has been a matter of growing concern for the last 150 years. This is not so much because attempts at control have failed, but rather that to some extent they have been successful. Many advances in modern medicine became possible only after infection was controlled. The fact that infection is still a problem is a reflection of the rapid expansion of medical science. The end of this process is not in sight. New diagnostic and therapeutic technologies will continue to bring new challenges to the control of infection.

This is not the end of the story, for three reasons. First, most hospitals are deficient in their practice of infection control because they do not apply all that is known about it. Secondly, some practices are wasteful or unnecessary. All of them need to be reviewed from time to time to see if they still are, or ever were, effective and cost-effective. Thirdly, the approach to infection control is less scientific than it should be. More logic and less woolly thought would make it easier to identify and cut out useless rituals, and to avoid making new mistakes. Attention to these three elements ought to shape the future development of infection control. They will be examined in turn.

Defective practices

It is very common to find that people working in hospitals are ignorant of the scale of HAI, or even deny that it exists. When the importance of these infections is underestimated, action to prevent them is of low priority, or nothing may be done at all. Failure to keep abreast of developments in the control of infection is also common. This may be due to pressure of work, or the lack of information. Even when information is available, lack of essential basic knowledge may lead to its misinterpretation. All of these difficulties are widespread, and they may coexist. However, the most common problem by far is the lack of resources. In a ward where there is no handbasin, or if no soap or towels are provided, calls for hand hygiene fall on deaf ears.

The scientific practice of infection control has developed in a spasmodic manner, based to a large extent on individual initiatives. Too often it is diluted by exhortation based on intuitive reasoning and degraded by erroneous ideas from the past. A considerable body of misinformation is the result. The proliferation of independant vocational groups within the health field has not helped. Groups that have sought and gained professional autonomy have, of course, exercised their right to educate new recruits to their ranks. Misplaced professional pride has sometimes led to unhealthy inbreeding among the educators appointed from within these groups.

The growth of knowledge in medicine is such that nobody can grasp all of it. Training in appropriate scientific disciplines is needed by those who are to interpret or evaluate developments within specialized fields. To understand the control of infection requires competence in epidemiology, infectious diseases and microbiology. To this basic information those who teach infection control need to add access to current literature in the field, and time to read and digest it. Even if non-specialist teachers can find the time and the motivation to read specialist textbooks on infection control, like all textbooks these are already out of date on the day they are published. Vocational groups among health-care workers are taught about the control of infection secondarily to the core subject of their speciality. Their teachers may be experts in the latter, but are unlikely to be so in the former. If they do not call on specialists in infection control or have no access to them, they may unwittingly use sources that are unreliable. In this way, error is perpetuated in the absence of the critical insight necessary to recognize that this is happening.

The same difficulty affects those members of the various professions who move into management. There they make decisions that decide policy. Where these decisions impinge on infection control, mistakes may be made by those whose knowledge of the subject depends on, perhaps, imperfect recollection of erroneous teaching received many years ago. It is only necessary to walk round new hospitals to see the unfortunate errors the more senior of such people can make. Infection control pervades many administrative matters in hospitals, usually as secondary or tertiary considerations. Managers and administrators who are perfectly able to make the primary decisions need to be aware of their limitations in these secondary areas. If they do not turn to the right quarter for the necessary advice, they are likely to make surprisingly expensive errors.

It has been suggested elsewhere (Chapter 3, p. 57) that in a perfect world each doctor and nurse would know enough about infection control to make specialist CIOs and ICNs redundant. This state of perfection will not be achieved for a long time, if ever. In the meantime, the deficiencies noted will be dealt with most efficiently by education, both initially and in service. This should involve all professional groups, not forgetting the educators themselves. Well-trained CIOs and ICNs are the primary resources in this respect. The skills required by these people are described in Chapter 3 (p. 49). Formal training courses for ICNs have been set up in many places. These should always be run by multi-disciplinary teachers to avoid the unhealthy inbreeding mentioned above. Because specialist knowledge to the level required is unlikely to be taught in ordinary nurse-training programmes, this is particularly important. Most of the training of CIOs is done by apprenticeship to an established practitioner. Short courses for CIOs are available in some countries. Again these are essential if inbreeding is to be avoided.

Cost effectiveness

A recurring theme in this book has been the need to question what is done to control infection to see if the practices are soundly based, or if some of them might be modified or abandoned to save money and resources. The object of infection control is to reduce morbidity and mortality in hospitals as much as possible, without wasting money. There is a long way to go before the first of these objectives is achieved, and even further for the second. Practices vary enormously between hospitals. Every ICT and ICC needs to review the rates of infection in their hospital and examine what is being done to control it. They are likely to find areas where they ought to do better (for example, in the use and care of urinary catheters) and locate pointless and expensive rituals (the over-use of disinfectants or unnecessary elaboration in dressing wounds, for instance). These monitoring activities will keep infection controllers busy for a long time.

The scientific approach

Infection control resembles a stool with three legs. The legs are epidemiology, infectious diseases and microbiology. Without all three the stool will fall over, and it will not provide a firm seat if any one leg is defective.

As Semmelweis showed (Chapter 1, p. 4) when epidemiology plus some knowledge of infectious diseases are properly applied, problems can be solved. The difficulty with this approach is that the detective work necessary takes time, years in Semmelweis' case. Where the unit of measurement is death, this time is expensive in human life. It is interesting to speculate what would have happened if Semmelweis had been able to call on microbiology to help him. This ought to have made his task easier and saved many lives. On the other hand, he might have been diverted from his epidemiological approach when he found (as he would have done) that the environment in his wards were hopping with streptococci. This happened to those bacteriologists in the 1930s who failed to be rigorous in their epidemiological thinking (Chapter 1, p. 7). The result was a waste of money that in some cases still continues.

The story of legionnaires' disease (legionellosis) is an example of the unavailing nature of epidemiology in the absence of microbiology. It was not possible to make the epidemiological facts of the famous Philadelphia outbreak mean anything until *Legionella pneumophila* had been isolated and its habits elucidated. The isolation took about six months to achieve, and much is now known about its habits. At a much more mundane level, the need to distinguish between clinically indistinguishable infections due to different bacteria, or that are caused by different types of the same one (Chapter 2, p. 26) underlines the total interdependence of epidemiology and microbiology. Because a study must start with an accurate definition, the third leg (a knowledge of infectious diseases) is also critical to a successful outcome.

If three people are required to provide the three forms of expertise, then there are six points of interpersonal contact at which communication can fail or friction develop. Other things being equal, and for economy, the smaller the number of people who are needed to bring together the three skills, the better. However, anyone who wishes to practice infection control effectively must recognize the importance of balancing this triple relationship. If less than three people are involved, care must be taken to see that one or more of the legs of the stool are not underdeveloped. A medical approach to disease is helpful. Microbiology without epidemiology will get nowhere, and epidemiology on its own will produce masses of data of little or no value. Only so much information should be collected as can be put to good use, either in the education of people so they behave better, or to act as the basis for properly designed studies of the causes or prevention of infection. If too much time is spent collecting data, there may be no time left to use them. If they are collected only for use in litigation, this is a sad comment on the modern practice of medicine.

It is clear that there is enormous potential for development in infection control. This will be achieved if practitioners base their activities firmly in science, though without forgetting their humanity.

Nothing is more caring than the control of infection, but this should depend on logical persuasion rather than on flights of the imagination and rhetorical exhortation. Most people know that windy rhetoric often conceals an intellectual void.

Appendix

DEFINITIONS OF INFECTIONS

A first and essential part of an epidemiological study is a careful definition of the phenomenon concerned (Chapter 2, p. 37). The reason for this is that if phenomena not related to the one being surveyed are included in a collection of data, they will confuse the analysis and may defeat the object. For example, early workers studying patients with yellow fever in South America were misled because cases of leptospirosis were inadvertently included, as both caused jaundice. The result was that the wrong conclusion was drawn, and a lot of time, effort and money was wasted. The definition of yellow fever they used did not exclude leptospirosis.

The study of HAI is a part of epidemiology, and so definitions are an essential starting point. Without definitions, surveys done by different people in the same hospital cannot be compared and, of course , recommendations made as the result of work done in one hospital or country cannot be transplanted without fear of error. The warning against including some pears when counting apples applies with great force when studying HAI.

If this were the only difficulty, the rest would be easy. Unfortunately, it is difficult to define infections. If this were not so, there would be no need of the many textbooks on infectious diseases and microbiology, some of which run into thousands of pages. Specialists in these subjects would not have to spend years learning just the basis of their crafts. Even experts in the field sometimes disagree. With HAI there are three more difficulties. First, if nurses or other paramedical staff are to collect raw data on hospital infections, they need clear, unambiguous instructions on how to interpret what they find. Secondly, they must be helped to make the often difficult distinction between colonization and infection (Chapter 2, p. 14). Thirdly, because it influences what is required, it must be clear who is to use the definitions drawn up, how they will use them, and for what purpose. It is not easy to distil the information available into a usable document. The result is not likely to please everybody.

A set of definitions may occupy a single sheet or occupy many pages. A fuller example comes from CDC Atlanta (Garner, J. S. *et al.* (1988). CDC definitions for nosocomial infections, 1988. *American*

Journal of Infection Control, **16**, 128–40). These are detailed and require careful study. Individuals using them would need to refer to them often until they became familiar. Presumably, because hospitals in the USA vary in size and the range of diagnostic facilities available to them, many of the definitions offer rather complex alternatives. At the other extreme are the very brief definitions used in the national survey of HAI conducted in England and Wales in 1980 (Meers, P. D. *et al.* (1981). Report on the national survey of infection in hospitals, 1980. *Journal of Hospital Infection*, **2**, Supplement, 48–51). These were prepared for use by individual teams in each of the 43 hospitals surveyed. The teams consisted of the hospital's CIO (usually a medically qualified microbiologist), an ICN and a senior nurse from each ward as it was surveyed. One member had been trained for the task beforehand, and a team, sometimes accompanied by an external scrutineer, visited each of the 18 186 patients involved. The definitions used are given below in a modified form to make them more generally applicable.

As with most choices concerned with infection control, local decisions about definitions are best made by the ICC of the hospital that needs them. They ought to take account of previous definitions, modifying these as necessary to suit their requirements (Chapter 2, p. 37). The way they are written must reflect the background training of the person or persons who are to use them.

Criteria for diagnosing an infection

1. In an **infection** the patient is reacting clinically or subclinically to the presence of a pathogenic microbe; if there is no reaction its presence is a **colonization**.
2. A **hospital acquired infection** is an infection found in a patient in hospital that was not present and was not being incubated on admission, or having been acquired in hospital, appeared after discharge. (This definition may be expanded to include infections in hospital employees that result from their employment.)
3. A **self-infection** is an infection due to a microbe that was part of the colonizing or normal flora of the patient before it appeared. Where this was present on the patient before admission to hospital, the infection is an **endogenous** self-infection. When the colonization is with a hospital pathogen and took place after admission, it is **autogenous** self-infection.
4. A **cross-infection** is an infection due to a microbe that originated from another patient or a member of staff in the hospital.
5. An **environmental infection** is an infection due to a microbe that originated in the environment of the patient.

6. **Urinary tract infection**: where the patient is being treated for a microbiologically or clinically diagnosed infection, or in whom a microbiological diagnosis has been made without treatment being given.

7. **Respiratory tract infection**:
   (a) **Upper**, where the patient has acute coryzal symptoms, or a significant sore mouth, throat, sinus or middle ear, not due to allergy.
   (b) **Lower**, where there is new or increased purulent sputum production with chest signs and (OR) X-ray changes not attributable to non-infectious causes.

8. **Wound infection**: a wound is a break in an epithelial surface (skin or mucous membrane) made by some act, such as an accident, burn or a surgical incision. Infected ulcers and pressure sores may be included under skin infections. A wound is infected if there is a purulent discharge in, or exuding from, it. (Infections may be classified as **minor** if the integrity of the wound is not threatened, or **major** if the wound seems likely to break down, or has done so.)

   In studying surgical wound infections, it is useful to categorize them as follows:
   (a) **Clean**, a surgical incision into non-inflamed tissue, when the gastrointestinal, respiratory or genital tracts are not entered.
   (b) **Clean-contaminated**, an otherwise clean wound which entered one of the above systems, where bacterial contamination might occur, but where no significant spillage was observed or was likely.
   (c) **Contaminated**, where one of the above systems has been opened and bacterial contamination is probable, or where inflammation is encountered.
   (d) **Dirty**, where pus is encountered, a perforated viscus found, or operations on contaminated traumatic wounds.

9. **Skin infection**: skin conditions demonstrating the classical signs of inflammation in skin and subcutaneous tissues.

10. (a) **Bacteraemia**: positive blood cultures, excluding those due to contamination, without symptoms.
    (b) **Septicaemia**: as above, and (OR) with symptoms of generalized sepsis.

11. **Infections of ears, eyes, genital tract**: significant new purulent discharge.

12. **CNS infections**: a positive culture from, or microscopy of, cerebrospinal fluid. Signs of an abscess or encephalitis.

13. **Gastrointestinal infection**:
    (a) **Generalized**, symptoms, plus a report of the recognition of

a gastrointestinal pathogen, or characteristic symptoms in an outbreak.

(b) **Localized**, a clinical diagnosis of appendicitis, diverticulitis, cholecystitis, anorectal sepsis, dental abscess, etc.

14. **Infections of bones and joints**: evidence of osteomyelitis or septic arthritis.

15. **Other infections**: any other obvious infection, including classical ones such as measles and hepatitis.

Index

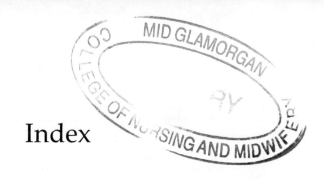